西部精神医学协会
Western China Psychiatric Association

临床躯体症状的心身医学分类及诊疗共识

Consensus for Psychosomatic Classification, Diagnosis and Treatment of Somatic Symptoms

第 2 版

孙学礼　曾凡敏　著
Editors: Xueli Sun　Fanmin Zeng

U0263212

科学出版社
北　京

内 容 简 介

躯体症状是引导患者就诊的主要因素，也是对患者造成直接痛苦并影响患者社会功能的主要原因。按现行的医学理念则将症状归入"疾病"系统，而对症状本身未给予充分重视。本"共识"是在 2015 年"共识"基础上的深入。本书的内容基于心身医学的理论框架，从生物、心理及社会多方面系统认识、分析、研究临床躯体症状，并从多个纬度探索其治疗规律。书中提出了躯体症状的心身分类，并在此假说的基础上修订了躯体症状的分类工具，展示了 2015～2016 年在国内近 80 家医疗单位开展的诊疗研究中运用假说、运用分类工具以及治疗各类躯体症状的进一步结果。

本书对医学界树立"大医学"理念及临床对躯体症状的综合识别与治疗有益，适合临床医师、护理人员以及医院管理者和广大医学生参考使用。

图书在版编目(CIP)数据

临床躯体症状的心身医学分类及诊疗共识/孙学礼，曾凡敏著. —2 版. —北京：科学出版社，2016.12

ISBN 978-7-03-051023-5

Ⅰ. 临… Ⅱ.①孙… ②曾… Ⅲ. 心身医学 Ⅳ.R395.1

中国版本图书馆 CIP 数据核字(2016)第 289534 号

责任编辑：丁慧颖 杨小玲 / 责任校对：李 影
责任印制：徐晓晨 / 封面设计：陈 敬

科 学 出 版 社 出版
北京东黄城根北街 16 号
邮政编码：100717
http://www.sciencep.com

北京虎彩文化传播有限公司 印刷
科学出版社发行 各地新华书店经销
*
2015 年 6 月第 一 版　开本：A5 (890×1240)
2017 年 1 月第 二 版　印张：6 1/2
2018 年 3 月第五次印刷　字数：158 000

定价：29.00 元
(如有印装质量问题，我社负责调换)

《临床躯体症状的心身医学分类及诊疗共识》
著作委员会

（按姓氏汉语拼音为序）

阿茹晗（四川大学华西临床医学院）

敖　天（成都肛肠专科医院便秘科）

毕　波（中国医科大学第一附属医院心理科）

陈　蕾（四川大学华西医院神经内科）

陈佳佳（成都市第四人民医院心身科）

代小松（四川省人民医院老年消化科）

戴光明（重庆市第三军医大学新桥医院神经内科）

邓美英（西安交通大学医学院第一附属医院神经内科）

董　强（四川大学华西医院泌尿外科）

董碧蓉（四川大学华西医院老干科）

杜　鹃（核工业部 416 医院神经内科）

段宝霖（青海省人民医院疼痛科）

段劲峰（绵阳市中心医院神经内科）

段志军（大连医科大学附属第一医院）

冯　杰（攀枝花市第三人民医院精神科）

冯志松（川北医学院附属医院消化内科）

高成阁（西安交通大学医学院第一附属医院精神科）

耿　婷（四川大学华西医院心理卫生中心）

龚文敬（成都肛肠专科医院便秘科）

谷姗姗（第三军医大学西南医院心身科）

郭　菁（四川大学华西临床医学院）

何　影（四川省人民医院心身科）

洪　军（南方医科大学南方医院心理科）

黄庆玲（第三军医大学大坪医院神经内科）

姜凤英（首都医科大学宣武医院神经内科）

况　利（重庆医科大学附属第一医院精神科）

李　南（重庆医科大学附属第一医院疼痛科）

李　伟（成都市第三人民医院神经内科）

李　懿（四川省人民医院消化内科）

李洪毅（成都市第四人民医院神经内科）

李会仓（宝鸡市中医医院神经内科）

李惠春（浙江大学医学院附属第二医院精神科）

李建阳（宁波市第二医院）

李劲梅（四川大学华西医院神经内科）

李良平（四川省人民医院消化科）

李苏宜（安徽省肿瘤医院肿瘤放疗科）

李晓裔（贵州省人民医院神经电生理科）

李幼辉（郑州大学附属第一医院精神科）

李云歌（成都市第四人民医院心身科）

廖宗炳（四川大学华西临床医学院）

刘　敏（青岛大学附属医院神经内科）

刘　平（德阳市人民医院神经内科）

刘　阳（四川大学华西医院心理卫生中心）

刘璨璨（四川大学华西临床医学院）

刘德良（中南大学湘雅二医院消化科）

刘铁桥（中南大学湘雅二医院心理科）

刘晓加（南方医科大学南方医院神经内科）

刘中霖（中山大学孙逸仙纪念医院神经内科）

卢　伟（郑州大学第一附属医院耳鼻喉科）

罗　娟（昆明医科大学第一附属医院消化科）

罗　云（达州中西医结合医院消化科）

梅　妍（天津医科大学总医院）

梅元武（华中科技大学同济医学院附属协和医院神经内科）

米　琛（西安交通大学第一附属医院消化科）

潘小平（广州市第一人民医院神经内科）

瞿　伟（重庆西南医院神经内科）

任　玲（四川大学华西医院康复科）

商慧芳（四川大学华西医院神经内科）

宿长军（第四军医大学唐都医院神经内科）

孙学礼（四川大学华西医院心理卫生中心）

谭友果（自贡市精神卫生中心）

陶　明（浙江省新华医院临床心理科）

田玉玲（山西医科大学第一医院神经内科）

王　浩（河南省人民医院高血压科）

王　琳（第三军医大学大坪医院神经内科）

王　荣（宿州市第一人民医院）

王　瑛（上海交通大学医学院附属瑞金医院神经内科）

王德燧（广元市精神卫生中心心身科）

王冠军（青岛市立医院心理科）

王化宁（第四军医大学西京医院心身科）

王庆松（成都军区总医院神经内科）

王艺明（贵阳医学院第一附属医院心理科）

吴薇莉（西华大学心理健康服务与研究中心）

吴孝苹（成都市第一人民医院神经内科）

武文珺（第四军医大学西京医院心身科）

熊小强（中山大学孙逸仙纪念医院消化科）

徐　理（四川省人民医院心身科）

徐佳军（四川大学华西医院心理卫生中心）

许秀峰（昆明医科大学第一附属医院精神科）

杨　蓓（云南省第二人民医院心内科）

杨　杰（成都市第一人民医院消化科）

杨　昆（绵阳市第三人民医院心身科）

杨邦祥（四川大学华西医院疼痛科）

杨才弟（四川省医学科学院附属医院神经内科）

杨东东（成都中医药大学附属医院神经内科）

杨小军（重庆中医院/重庆市中医研究院脾胃科）

杨晓秋（重庆医科大学附属第一医院疼痛科）

杨晓昀（鄂尔多斯市中心医院）

杨彦春（四川大学华西医院心理卫生中心）

杨志秀（云南省第二人民医院神经内科）

易智慧（四川大学华西医院消化内科）

余　琴（西南医科大学附属医院心内科）

余能伟（四川省人民医院神经内科）

喻小念（北京航空总医院心身科）

袁亦铭（北京大学第一医院男科）

曾　仲（成都市第三人民医院神经内科）

曾凡敏（西南民族大学社会学与心理学学院）

查定军（第四军医大学西京医院耳鼻喉科）

詹淑琴（首都医科大学宣武医院神经内科）

郑　毅（首都医科大学附属北京安定医院）

张　欢（西安交通大学医学院第二附属医院精神心理科）

张颖慧（四川省人民医院消化科）

张震中（新疆维吾尔自治区中医医院脑病科）

周　波（四川省人民医院心身科）

周　焱（四川大学华西医院老干科）

周冀英（重庆医科大学附属第一医院神经内科）

周晓晴（南充市中心医院消化科）

周亚玲（四川大学华西临床医学院）

朱润秀（内蒙古自治区人民医院神经内科）

邹开庆（雅安市第三人民医院心身科）

邹晓毅（成都上锦南府医院-华西上锦分院神经内科）

The Committee (in Chinese Phonetic Alphabets Order of Surnames)

Ruhan A (West China School of Medical, Sichuan University)

Tian Ao (The Department of Constipation of Chengdu Anorectal Hospital)

Bo Bi (The Department of Psychology of the First Hospital of China Medical University)

Jiajia Chen (The Department of Psychosomatic Medicine of The Fourth People's Hospital Chengdu)

Lei Chen (The Department of Neurology of West China Hospital, Sichuan University)

Guangming Dai(The Department of Neurology of Xinqiao Hospital, Third Military Medical Universit)

Xiaosong Dai (The Department of geriatric Gastroenterology of Sichuan Provincial People's Hospital)

Meiying Deng (The Department of Neurology of the First Affiliated Hospital of Xi'an Jiaotong University)

Qiang Dong (The Department of Urology of West China Hospital, Sichuan University)

Birong Dong (The Department of Geriatric Medicine of West China Hospital, Sichuan University)

Juan Du (The Department of Neurology of the Nuclear Industry 416 Hospital)

Baolin Duan (The Department of Pain Medicine of Qinghai Provincial People's Hospital)

Jinfeng Duan (The Department of Neurology of Mianyang Central Hospital)

Zhijun Duan (The First Affiliated Hospital of Dalian Medical University)

Jie Feng (The Department of Psychiatry of the Third People's Hospital of Panzhihua)

Zhisong Feng (The Department of Gastroenterology of Affiliated Hospital of North Sichuan Medical College)

Chengge Gao (The Department of Psychiatry of the First Affiliated Hospital of Xi'an Jiaotong University)

Ting Geng (The Mental Health Center of West China Hospital, Sichuan University)

Wenjing Gong (The Department of Constipation of Chengdu Anorectal Hospital)

Shanshan Gu (The Department of Psychosomatic Medicine of South West Hospital in the Third Military Medical University)

Jing Guo (West China School of Medical, Sichuan University)

Ying He (The Department of Psychosomatic Medicine of Sichuan Provincial People's Hospital)

Jun Hong (The Department of Psychology of Nanfang Hospital of Southern Medical University)

Qingling Huang (The Department of Neurology of DaPing Hospital of the Third Military Medical University)

Fengying Jiang (The Department of Neurology of Xuanwu Hospital Capital Medical)

Li Kuang (The Department of Psychiatry of the First Affiliated Hospital of Chongqing Medical University)

Nan Li (The Department of Pain Medicine of the First Affiliated Hospital of Chongqing Medical University)

Hongyi Li (The Department of Neurology of The Fourth People's Hospital Chengdu)

Huicang Li (The Department of Neurology of Baoji City Chinese Medicine Hospital)

Huichun Li（The Department of Psychiatry of The Second Affiliated Hospital of Zhejiang University School of Medical）

Jianyang Li (The Second Hospital of Ningbo City)

Jinmei Li (The Department of Neurology of West China Hospital, Sichuan University)

Liangping Li（The Department of Gastroenterology of Sichuan Provincial People's Hospital）

Suyi Li (The Department of Radiotherapy of Anhui Provincial Cancer Hospital)

Wei Li (The Department of Neurology of The Third People's Hospital of Chengdu)

Xiaoyi Li (The Department of Neuroelectrophysiology of Guizhou Provincial People's Hospital)

Yi Li (The Department of Psychosomatic Medicine of Sichuan Provincial

People's Hospital)

Youhui Li (The Department of Psychiatry of the First Affiliated Hospital of Zhengzhou University)

Yunge Li（The Department of Psychosomatic Medicine of The Fourth People's Hospital Chengdu）

Zongbing Liao (West China School of Medical, Sichuan University)

Cancan Liu (West China School of Medical, Sichuan University)

Deliang Liu (The Department of Gastroenterology of the Second Xiangya Hospital of Central South University)

Min Liu (The Department of Neurology of the Affiliated Hospital of Qingdao University)

Ping Liu (The Department of Neurology of People's Hospital of Deyang City)

Tieqiao Liu (The Department of Psychology of the Second Xiangya Hospital of Central South University)

Xiaojia Liu (The Department of Neurology of Nanfang hospital of Southern Medical University)

Yang Liu (The Mental Health Center of West China Hospital, Sichuan University)

Zhonglin Liu (The Department of Neurology of Sun Yat-sen Memorial Hospital, Sun Yat-sen University)

Wei Lu (The Department of Otolaryngology of the First Affiliated Hospital of Zhengzhou University)

Juan Luo (The Department of Gastroenterology of First Affiliated Hospital of Kuming Medical University)

Yun Luo (The Department of Gastroenterology of Dazhou Hospital of Integrated Traditional And Western Medicine)

Yan Mei (Tianjin Medical University General Hospital)

Yuanwu Mei (The Department of Neurology of Wuhan Union Hospital Tongji Medical College, Huazhong University of Science And Technology)

Chen Mi (The Department of Gastroenterology of the First Affiliated Hospital of Xi'an Jiaotong University)

Xiaoping Pan (The Department of Neurology of The First People's Hospital of Guangzhou)

Wei Qu (The Department of Neurology of South West Hospital)

Ling Ren (Rehabilitation Medical Center, West China Hospital, Sichuan University)

Huifang Shang (The Department of Neurology of West China Hospital, Sichuan University)

Changjun Su (The Department of Neurology of Tangdu Hospital of the Fourth Military Medical University)

Xueli Sun (The Mental Health Center of West China Hospital, Sichuan University)

Ming Tao (The Department of clinical psychology of Xinhua Hospital in Zhejiang Province)

Youguo Tan (The Department of Psychiatry of Zigong Mental Health Center)

Yuling Tian (The Department of Neurology of The First Affiliated Hospital of ShanXi Medical University)

Desui Wang (The Department of Psychosomatic Medicine of Guangyuan Mental Health Center Four Hospital)

Guanjun Wang (The Department of Psychology of Qingdao Municipal Hospital)

Hao Wang (The Department of Hypertension of Henan Provincal People's Hospital)

Huaning Wang (The Department of Psychosomatic Medicine of Xijing Hospital of the Fourth Military Medical University)

Lin Wang (The Department of Neurology of Daping Hospital, Research Institute of Surgery Third Military Medical University)

Qingsong Wang (The Department of Neurology of Chengdu Military General Hospital)

Rong Wang (First People's Hospital of Suzhou City)

Yiming Wang (The Department of Psychology of Affiliated Hospital of Guiyang Medical College)

Ying Wang (The Department of Neurology of Rui Jin Hospital Shanghai Jiao Tong University School of Medicine)

Xiaoping Wu (The Department of Neurology of Chengdu First People's Hospital)

Weili Wu (Mental Health Services and Research Center of Xiha University)

Wenjun Wu (The Department of Psychosomatic Medicine of Xijing Hospital)

Xiaoqiang Xiong (The Department of Gastroenterology of Sun Yat-sen Memorial Hospital, Sun Yat-sen University)

Jiajun Xu (The Mental Health Center of West China Hospital, Sichuan University)

Li Xu (The Department of Psychosomatic Medicine of Sichuan Provincial People's Hospital)

Xiufeng Xu(The Department of Psychiatry of First Hospital Affilicated to Kunming Medical University)

Bangxiang Yang (The Department of Pain Medicine of West China Hospital, Sichuan University)

Caidi Yang (The Department of Neurology of Affiliated Hospital of Sichuan Academy of Medical Sciences)

Dongdong Yang (The Department of Neurology of Teaching Hospital of Chengdu University of T.C.M)

Jie Yang (The Department of Gastroenterology of Chengdu First People's Hospital)

Kun Yang (The Department of Psychosomatic Medicine of the Third Hospital of Mianyang)

Xiaoyun Yang (Ordos Central Hospital)

Xiaojun Yang (The Department of Gastroenterology of Chongqing Traditional Chinese Medical Hospital)

Yanchun Yang (The Mental Health Center of West China Hospital, Sichuan University)

Xiaoqiu Yang (The Department of Pain Medicine of the First Affiliated Hospital of Chongqing Medical University)

Zhixiu Yang (The Department of Neurology of the Second People's Hospital of Yunnan Province)

Zhihui Yi (The Department of Gastroenterology of West China Hospital, Sichuan University)

Nengwei Yu (The Department of Neurology of Sichuan Provincial People's Hospital)

Qin Yu (The Department of Cardiology of the Affiliated Hospital of Southwest Medical University)

Xiaonian Yu (The Department of Psychosomatic Medicine of Aviation General Hospital of China Medical University)

Yiming Yuan (Peking University First Hospital Andrology Center)

Dingjun Zha (The Department of Otolaryngology of Xijing Hospital of the Fourth Military Medical University)

Huan Zhang (The Department of Psychology and Psychiatry of the Second Affiliated Hospital of Xi'an Jiaotong University)

Yinghui Zhang (The Department of Gastroenterology of Sichuan Provincial People's Hospital)

Zhenzhong Zhang (The Department of Encephalopathy Medicine of Hospital of Chinese Medicine of the Xinjiang Uygur Autonomous Region)

Zhong Zeng (The Department of Neurology of The Third People's Hospital of Chengdu)

Fanmin Zeng (The School of Sociology and Psychology in Southwest University for Nationalities)

Suqin Zhan (The Department of Neurology of Xuanwu Hospital Capital Medical University)

Yi Zheng (Beijing Anding Hospital of Capital Medical University)

Bo Zhou (The Department of Psychosomatic Medicine of Sichuan provincial people's hospital)

Yaling Zhou (West China School of Medical, Sichuan University)

Yan Zhou (The Department of Geriatric Medicine of West China Hospital, Sichuan University)

Xiaoqing Zhou (The Department of Gastroenterology of Nanchong Central Hospital)

Jiying Zhou (The Department of Neurology of The First Affiliated Hospital of Chongqing Medical University)

Runxiu Zhu (The Department of Neurology of Inner Mongolia Autonomous Region People's Hospital)

Kaiqing Zou (The Department of Psychosomatic Medicine of The Third People's Hospital of Yaan)

Xiaoyi Zou (The Department of Neurology of Cheng Du Shang Jin Nan Fu Hospital West China Hospital, S.C.U)

序

当医疗机构面临众多患者的时候，临床医护人员都忙于诊断、治疗和护理。但是否思考过这样的问题：是什么因素促进患者的就诊？总结医疗机构收治患者的情况，促进患者就诊的因素无非有二：一是由于偶然因素或定期体检发现躯体出现某些病理变化，而这些"变化"经以往研究或临床实践证明可以给个体带来严重后果，甚至危及生命，如恶性肿瘤，所以尽管目前当事人没有丝毫不适感觉，但也要就诊并积极治疗，此时治疗的意义实际上是对未来可能出现的危险甚至危及生命的情况的预防；二是由于个体出现各种躯体不适的情况，即各种躯体症状，而这些躯体症状对个体的生活质量，正常工作、学习构成影响，因而就诊，此时就诊及接受治疗的目的是改善自身的不良感受。而实际工作中发现，后一类就诊情况占大多数，也就是说，我们面对的真正的当下的患者是带着躯体症状来寻求医疗援助的个体，由此医学领域关注、研究及诊治临床症状顺理成章。

但医学界目前的问题是习惯将千姿百态的临床症状归入已经界定的疾病中，换句话讲，就是医学关注"疾病"或关注可查见的病理损害重于关注症状。建立这一诊疗理念是基于"症状是由疾病或可查见的病理损害引起的，治愈疾病或消除病理损害后症状自然消失"的认识。但前述认识存在问题，其一是疾病的界定，严格意义上讲，疾病是一个社会学概念而非医学概念，其意义在于为社保、劳动能力界定、家庭看护等提供依据。当然，疾病的界定对于确定医学的工作范围，以及专门技术的发展也同样有意义。医学界对疾病概念有过长期的讨论。有人认为病理损害应该称为疾病，但反对者认为有的病理损害或病理改变不具疾病特征，也不能称为疾病，如"鸡眼"；又有人提出个体感到痛苦称为疾病，但反对者认为痛苦情况很多，如失恋、过度劳累等。此外，精神病学中被医学界明确界定为疾病的躁狂症，患者比正常时的体验还愉快，基于这些情况，痛苦等于疾病的说法被否定。目前医学界对疾病的界定实际上是基于对健康概念的延伸。众所周知，生理、心理、社会的完满状态被视为健康，而不完满状态理应被视为亚健康，而当这种亚健康状态达到影响个体的社会功能或给本人带来严重痛苦时（精神或躯体），便将这种情况视为医学应予以干预的亚健康状态，即"疾病"。据此可以认为，医学领域所称的"疾病"是一个连续的过程，而非一种静止的状态。例如，某些糖代谢指标超过一定范围被称为"糖耐量异常"，当这种异常达到一定程度，便称为"糖尿病"，而再由此进一步发展，就可以出现皮肤、肾脏、血管、心脏等多器官损害，而随着上述过程的发展，医学介入的范围会越来越深、越来越广。从以上对疾病的思考可以认为，重视病理生理或病理心理过程是为了阻止将来危险情况的发生，而重视患者的躯体症状是为了缓解患者目前的痛苦，两者同样重要。此外，充足理由律提示，前提与结论之间必须存在必然的逻辑联系，躯体症状是不愉快的主观体验，既然是"主观体验"，就必然与心理、社会等多元因素相关，而非仅与"损伤"或"潜在损伤"相关。因而，仅仅关注"损伤"或"潜在损伤"就不可能很好地解决躯体症状给个体带来的痛苦，也就达不到治疗"当下"患者的目的。因此，从心理、生理及社会诸方面系统地认识、分析、研究临床躯体症状，并从多个维度探索其治疗规律成为必要。

　　基于以上原因，西部精神医学协会 2014 年设立了相关项目，提出了躯体症状的心身医学定义、分类假说，并在此假说的基础上制订了相应的分类工具，并在 2015 年出版了运用假说及制订的分类工具在国内近 70 家医疗单位开展的诊疗研究所得到的初步结果。新的理念需要不断地丰富和完善，同时自然条件下所形成的"优化治疗方案"也需要在不断扩大治疗样本的基础上得到认定。因此，国内近 80 家医疗单位在 2015～2016 年近 1 年的时间内继续在躯体症状心身医学分类理念基础上进行临床实践,得到了 2016 年的"共识"。本"共识"较 2014～2015 年的"共识"在躯体症状的心身医学分类、躯体症状分类量表,以及优化治疗方面都有一些新的变化,可供参考。还是那句话,希望能够对医学界树立"大医学"的理念及医学临床对躯体症状的综合识别与治疗有所贡献。认识是不断发展的,本"共识"也需被不断完善和证伪,因此欢迎来自不同地区、不同文化背景、不同国度的业内人士提出不同的意见并进一步贡献相关方面的实践资料从而达成更广范围的共识。

孙学礼

2016.8 于成都

Preface

Doctors and nurses are tied up with diagnosis, treatment and nursing care when facing the patients crowed in the waiting area. Here is the question: Why are there so many patients? Summary of patients admitted to the medical institutions, promoting factors in patients of no more than two: one is the incidental factors or regular physical examination found the body with certain pathological changes, and the previous study of the "change" or clinical practice has been proved that they can cause serious consequences for the individual, even life-threatening, such as malignant tumor. So even the patients did not have any discomfort, active treatment shall be given. The treatment in fact is crucial to prevent diseases or even life-threatening situation in the future; the other is the individually different physical discomfort, *i.e.* various somatic symptoms, influence of which on the quality of life, work or learning leads to the visit to the doctors. The diagnosis and treatment at this moment are to improve their ailments. But in clinical practice, this kind of treatment is in the majority, that is to say, the patients come to us just because they are physically ill, so followed by the medicinal attention, medical research and clinical diagnosis and treatment of symptoms.

However, the problem is that we always want classified these clinical symptoms into some kind of diseases, in other word, the physicians care more about the "disease" or observable pathological damage than clinical symptoms. Such medical philosophy is formed based on the misunderstanding of "symptoms are caused by disease or observable pathological damages, symptoms disappear naturally after the diseases are cured or pathological damages are eliminated". There are still problems needed to be solved, one of which is the definition of disease, which, technically, is a sociological concept rather than medical, its significance lies in providing the basis for the social security, the ability to work and family care. Of course, the definition of disease is also important to determine the scope of work and medical expertise. The medical industry has a very long discussion on concept of disease: first, some people think that the pathological damage should be referred to as the disease, but their opponents argue that some pathological damage or pathological changes with disease characteristics shall not be called disease, such as "corn". And some people think that physical pain is a disease, but the opponents say the pain can be induced under a lot of circumstances, such as being dumped or too tired; in addition, mania, a psychiatric term, which is also considered as a disease by the medical community, but oddly it is more enjoyable for a patient when experiencing a mania attack. So, we don't think it is right to hold the idea that pain equals disease. At present, the definition of disease, according to the consensus of the medical industry, is the extension of the concept of health. As everyone knows, the perfect state of physiological, psychological, social life is considered healthy, while those not should be regarded as sub-healthy, and when the sub-healthy state has an influence on the individual's social function or brings severe pain (mental or physical), then this kind of situation which need medical intervention can be called a "disease". It can be said, the definition "disease" is a continuous process, rather than a static state. For example, when carbonhydrate metabolism exceeding a certain range, is known as the "abnormal glucose tolerance", when this abnormality aggravates to a certain extent, it is called "diabetes", and then further development may inducing multiple organ failure involving the skin, kidney, blood vessels and heart, *etc.*

With the development of abovementioned process, the scope of medical intervention will be wider and wider, the degree of involvement will be deeper and deeper. It is thought, based on the above consideration of disease, paying attention to pathophysiological or pathopsychological process is important to prevent the diseases, and the focus on the symptom is to relieve the pain of patients, both are equally important. According to the law of sufficient reason, there must be a logical relationship between premises and conclusion, somatic symptoms are unpleasant experience, since it is a "subjective experience, it is associated with psychological, social and other factors, not only the "damage" or "potential damage". Therefore, only paying attention to "damage" or "potential damage" would not be a good solution to the individual physical symptoms of pain, it won't bring immediate pain remission to the patients. Therefore, it is necessary to study and analyze the disease from the psychological, physiological and social aspects and explore the treatment law from multiple dimensions.

Based on the above reasons, West China Psychiatry Association in 2014 set up the related project, and put forward the definition, classification of psychosomatic symptoms, and on the basis of the hypothesis formulated the corresponding classification tool, and show the preliminary results using the hypothesis and make classification tool in diagnosis and treatment carried out in nearly 70 domestic medical units in 2014. The new concepts need to constantly enrich and perfect, at same time the "optimization treatment" was formed by the natural conditions also need to sample expanded. So domestic nearly 80 medical units in 2015 and 2016, nearly 1 years of time to continue in the clinical practice of the somatic symptoms of psychosomatic medicine classification concept, formed the "consensus" in 2016. The new "consensus" from "consensus" in 2014-2015 in the somatic symptoms of psychosomatic medicine classification, the classification scale of the somatic symptoms and optimizing the treatment have some new changes, which for your reference. We hope to establish the idea of "medicine and clinical medicine" to contribute to the recognition and treatment of somatic symptoms. Knowledge is growing, the "consensus" also needs to be constantly improved and falsified. Therefore, different views from different regions, cultural backgrounds or countries are welcomed to contribute further to the relevant aspects of the practice so as to reach a broader consensus.

Xueli Sun

2016.8 Chengdu

目录/Contents

第一章　心身医学理论框架下临床躯体症状分类的相关问题

第一节　躯体症状分类的心身医学理论假说

临床医学各个学科都会面临患者的各种躯体症状。按照常规的临床思维模式，症状总是有相应的病理基础，因此躯体症状就成了提示各种躯体病理改变的线索，同时也成为启动诊断及治疗流程的基本依据。为了更好地执行上述的诊断及治疗过程，临床上将躯体症状按系统进行分类，如呼吸系统症状、消化系统症状、泌尿系统症状、心血管系统症状、神经系统症状等。这样就便于临床医师循着症状的线索进行分诊、对相应系统进行查体及实验室检查并规划治疗方案。这种传统的思维方式存在几个问题：其一，出现在某个系统的症状不一定就提示那个系统的问题，因此当循着症状在相应的系统发现不了问题的时候，诊疗活动就没法进行下去，而将患者转诊到其他学科则意味着诊疗活动的重新开始，从而浪费诊断资源及时间；其二，有的症状的归类存在重叠，因此很难将其定位在某一个系统，如可以将呕吐归为消化系统症状，也可将其归为神经系统症状，当按一个系统疾病治疗无效时，就只能改变治疗方向，这就意味着对某患者的治疗重新开始，从而浪费治疗资源及治疗时间；其三，"一个原因必然导致一个结果"，这是一元化思维模式，这种思维模式可以使临床思维绝对化、固定化和"标准化"，但事实上一个原因不止导致一种结果，反之一个结果可以由多个原因引起，缺乏多元化的思维模式，以及从多个角度去考虑一个问题的习惯必然会导致临床及科研思路的僵化，从而影响到对疾病的认识和治疗。例如，某患者下腹疼痛，月经失调，检查发现了子宫肌瘤，立刻行肌瘤切除手术，但事与愿违，术后患者疼痛加剧，甚至无法起床，几乎酿成医疗纠纷，经抗焦虑治疗 2~4 周后，患者疼痛消失，顺利出院并恢复工作。该案例说明，虽然症状出现在下腹部，但问题出在患者的精神方面，至少说明多方面原因共同导致患者的疼痛，而仅按一个系统的问题进行治疗必然得不到预期的结果。

　　临床上任何分类、诊断的目的都是为更有针对性地治疗，同时也是为临床诊疗提供正确的思路，而以上几点说明按系统来认识躯体症状的传统方式存在缺陷和误区。"躯体症状是与组织损伤和潜在损伤相关的不愉快的主观感觉"。这是目前临床上对躯体症状较为公认的定义，从该定义理解，躯体症状实质上是一种"感受"，而这种"感受"的产生既与"损伤"或"潜在损伤"有关，又与个体的体验有关。换一句话说，根据该定义的提示，任何躯体症状的产生都不是纯生物源性的，而总是与其认知、情感、个性等心理元素相关。基于这种思路，躯体症状还可以做如下解读。

一、躯体症状是躯体组织或器官对外界环境的述求

　　此定义来源于"述情理论"及"继发性获益理论"。要简要阐述这两个理论，又要涉及前面所提到的"无意识"。器官功能改变表达述求是生物界存在的普遍现象，如小动物因恐惧所出现的小便失禁、肌肉震颤，日常生活中常提到的"我见到你就恶心"等均是器官功能变化表达"述求"的例证。由于人神经系统的进化和发育，人类表达"述求"的主要方式是言语或情感，如果某个个体仍将器官功能变化病理基础作为表达"述求"的主要途径，这种情况就称为"述情障碍"。某 18 岁女性因严重呕吐 1 年之内住院 7 次，每次住院缓解迅速，但反复发作，实验室检查未发现导致呕吐的病理基础，了解成长过程及目前心态发现，该患者内心暗恋上了自己的亲哥哥，而呕吐应该是对自己这种情感的厌恶，经这种分析、心理疏导，以及辅以抗焦虑治疗，呕吐消失，追踪观察两年，呕吐未再出现。该案例是躯体症状作为"述

求"出现的最好说明。如果无意识地将自己的躯体功能障碍作为获得实际利益的"筹码",这种情况称为"继发性获益"。作为基于这一病理心理基础的转换障碍是最好的例证。

二、躯体症状是缓解内心冲突的重要途径

症状是躯体与心灵连接的桥梁,个体往往不能意识到自己深层的内心冲突,其代价是出现躯体症状,在与外界环境身心交瘁的搏斗中,最终躯体忍无可忍,不得不提出"抗议",当然这种抗议是隐秘的、是在潜意识水平的,转而表现为躯体症状,这样内心冲突就以比较能接受的躯体形式表达出来了,这样既不威胁到个体的自我形象。也保护了个体精神免遭崩溃,同时还"抗议"了现实生活压力。在这样的冲突中,患者无法直接表达他的冲突,只有通过躯体症状——象征性地把冲突吞下。一只狐狸走到葡萄架下想吃葡萄,但费了九牛二虎之力也没法爬上葡萄架,狐狸面临两种选择,一是拼命爬上去,这意味着要强迫自己继续干力所不能及的事情,二是放弃,这意味着要痛苦地承认自己的能力不够,而狐狸采取了自己所能接受的第三种方式,"葡萄是酸的,不吃了"。这是心理防卫机制合理化的最好说明。将这种情景换成一个不是优等生的学生希望能够取得优异成绩,对该学生也存在两种选择:一是努力达成第一名,这意味着他或她必须付出力所不能及的努力;二是放弃成为优等生的目标,这意味着他或她必须承认自己不是优等生,而解决这种内心冲突的途径就是"因为我病了,所以成为不了优等生",此时的躯体症状就成了缓解内心冲突的途径。

三、躯体症状就是情绪本身

既然躯体症状是"不愉快的主观体验",如果要将躯体症状定义为情绪本身,则这种情形显然是指的负性情绪。临床上常见的负性情绪主要是焦虑和抑郁。以焦虑为例,临床上对焦虑的解读是内心体验的不安或恐惧伴自主神经系统功能紊乱及运动不安,因此焦虑涉及躯

体层面、体验层面和认知层面。焦虑是人的基本情绪，焦虑的基本意义是使生物个体保持必要的警觉性，这和生物体的自我防御直接相关。提示警觉性增高及自我防卫的典型躯体症状是疼痛，此外，表现为器官功能混乱的症状或综合征，如尿频、尿急，肠易激综合征等。

四、躯体症状是个体对躯体感受的负性解读

该定义主要表明人的认知系统在躯体症状产生中的作用。各种感受随时存在，通过认知的影响，个体如果对某种感受做正性解读，就成为个体此时需要的感受，如果做负性解读，这种感受就成为个体需要排斥的感受，就成为躯体症状。再以疼痛为例，当将其作为负性解读的时候，疼痛成为最常见的临床症状之一，但人们有的时候也在追求疼痛的感觉，甚至觉得"爽"，如在接受保健按摩的时候，疼痛便不成为困扰个体的"症状"，而是此刻所寻求的正性感受。

五、躯体症状是学习或模仿的结果

该定义主要表明在暗示或自我暗示的情况下，个体可以再现以往的症状或复制别人的症状。所谓暗示是指在一定的环境下和一定的情感氛围中个体对来自外界的影响无条件接受的情况，而在一定的环境下和一定的情感氛围中对来自自身的影响无条件接受的情况称为自我暗示。暗示和自我暗示是人的心理特性，早期研究表明 5～7 岁暗示性最高，女性的暗示性高于男性，随着年龄增长，暗示性逐渐减弱。而随年龄增长，个体的暗示性仍然保持在与实际年龄不相符合时，这种暗示性就成为产生躯体症状的高危心理因素。在此种情况下，躯体症状所提示的问题不是躯体器官的病理损害而是异常的暗示性。此外，该定义还提示，未成年人、青壮年、老年出现同样症状的心理意义是不同的。

如果以上定义均成立，躯体症状的意义就不仅是提示躯体疾病，同时也可作为提示精神疾病、心理异常、个性特质的证据。

第二节 躯体症状心身分类的具体建议

根据对躯体症状的以上解读，患者，即使是某种躯体疾病的患者出现的躯体症状也应该存在两种成分，一种是"生物学成分"，如肿瘤病变所导致的躯体症状，而另一种成分在此暂时称为"心理成分"。采用心身医学理论来解读临床躯体症状所表明的问题是多元化的思维方式对临床工作的指导作用。医学上的惯性思维是一元化的思维模式，落实到具体问题上就是患者有躯体症状，临床医师总是仅从病理损害的角度去查找原因并给予相应的处理，而忽略了"心理成分"的存在，因而使患者的躯体症状得不到满意解决，而躯体症状的存在对患者的心态、生活质量、治疗依从性及预后都是至关重要的，值得注意。此外，充足理由律提示，前提与结论之间应存在必然的逻辑联系。有症状存在，同时有病理损害存在，因此就判断症状是病理损害的结果这种思维模式违背充足理由律，如果成为临床医学的惯性思维就值得反思。躯体症状的心身医学解读为全面分析躯体症状和分析不同个体所存在的同样症状提供了依据。那么，依照心身医学对躯体症状解读的观点，对慢性非感染疾病治疗至少有三个维度，一是病因学治疗维度，二是病理生理、病理心理治疗维度，三是症状学治疗维度。因此，对躯体症状的独立治疗应得到更多的关注。

为满足针对躯体症状独立治疗的需要，根据以上对躯体症状的解读，从心身医学的观点综合评价，躯体症状大致可以分类为以下情况。

一、生物性躯体症状

生物性躯体症状即主要由物理、化学、生物因素所产生的局部损伤直接导致的神经末梢刺激或由于局部组织损伤后的生化反应所导致的对神经末梢的次级刺激所产生的症状。该类症状产生的基础不是刺激的种类和强度，而应该是神经系统上行通路的激活，以及下传通路的脱抑制。值得注意的是，上行通路的激活与下传通路的脱抑制受阻不仅源于生物学的损害，也可源于，甚至更可源于心态的变化，如战斗或其他激情状态下，个体可以对由损伤所产生的疼痛毫无知觉。这说明即使是生物学损害，其是否产生躯体负性感受或产生什么样的感受与心理因素也密切相关。

二、情绪性躯体症状

在这种情况下，躯体症状本身就是负性情感的表现。根据"述情"理论，躯体症状是器官对外界环境的述求。一般情况下，这种"述求"见于负性情绪，常见的负性情绪主要是抑郁和焦虑，因此又可将"情绪"症状分为"抑制性情绪症状"和"激惹性情绪症状"。顾名思义，前者主要指的是躯体器官功能受到抑制的各种表现，如厌食、饱胀感、头昏、不清醒感等，最典型的抑制性躯体症状是功能性消化不良所表现出的症状；后者则是指局部激惹所表现的功能失调，如疼痛、肠易激综合征所表现出的症状。

三、认知性躯体症状

此处的"认知"有两个含义，一是指个体对躯体感知的"解读"。躯体的各种感受总是存在的，只有当个体在认知层面将某种"感受"做负性解读的时候，这种"感受"才能成为"躯体症状"。如当某个体疲劳后接受保健按摩的时候，很多人会要求力量重一点，从而获得舒服及放松的感觉，在这种情况下，疼痛是被需求的，在认知层面，此时的疼痛是被作"正性"解读的，而当疼痛被作为负性信息解读的时候就成了某种损伤的"预警信号"，也就成为躯体症状。精神病学对幻觉所下的定义是在没有客观刺激作用于感觉器官的情况下，在相应的感觉器官所出现的知觉体验，对照幻觉的定义可以发现，有的躯体症状符合幻觉的定义，这就是认知性躯体症状的第二层含义。例如，双侧具有知觉性质的耳鸣可以作为幻觉理解并作为幻觉治疗。认知性躯体症状的特征为症状的性质及部位相对固定，症状清晰、生动。例如，某中年女性患者以跛行入院，跛行的原因是行走时感到右足底像踩着一块较尖锐的约鸽蛋大小的鹅卵石，因此很痛，故而跛行。经采用非典型抗精神病药物治疗两周后症状消失。

四、想象性躯体症状

此处所指的"想象"就是患者的暗示或自我暗示所产生的症状，该类症状的特点应该是症状多变性及症状的"超常性"，如某青年女性患者曾多次发作性出现自己"脑细胞"一层层往下掉的感觉，并因此感到恐慌而急诊就医，在发作时可以清晰地描述一层层的脑细胞"掉"到膝关节、踝关节的情况。

以上对躯体症状分类的意义在于：首先，有利于拓展临床思路，并有利于在对躯体症状的理解中更好地贯彻心身统一的观点；其次，有利于从躯体症状的认识中寻求诊断躯体疾病及精神疾病的方向；再次，有利于确定对躯体症状的治疗方向，如对"抑制性症状"的抗抑郁治疗、对"激惹性症状"的抗焦虑治疗、对认知性症状的改善认知的药物和心理治疗、对生物性躯体症状的局部及全身病变的治疗等。值得注意的是，即使是从以上角度理解躯体症状也应因人而异和贯彻"多元化"的思维模式。例如，同样的疼痛可能是激惹性躯体症状，可能是认知性躯体症状，也可能是想象性的躯体症状，所以在对于具体患者的躯体症状性质的判断中应注意患者症状的组合、病史、生活经历、人格特征、情绪等因素。即使是对于局部损伤或潜在损伤所导致的生物性躯体症状的治疗也同样应注意上述非生物学因素。因为即使是在生物学病变存在的情况下，决定躯体症状存在的因素也绝非仅仅是生物学因素。例如，同样的损伤，有的患者疼痛仅持续几天，而有的患者则可存在数年。总之心身统一的观点，以及多元化的临床思维模式是认识躯体症状和治疗躯体症状的重要前提。

（孙学礼　著）

第二章 心身医学理论框架下临床躯体症状分类工具修订

第一节 《西部精神医学协会（WCPA）临床躯体症状分类量表》修订

在2014～2015年的现场测试中，我们收集了自编《西部精神医学协会（WCPA）临床躯体症状分类量表》使用反馈意见，主要体现在：①对情绪症状细分不明确；②没有体现出节律症状；③关于症状描述的语言表述不够规范。由于受采样现场和采样时间的限制，在2015～2016现场测试过程中，我们专门对反映情绪症状的条目进行了修改，强调了对情绪性躯体症状中激惹性躯体症状和抑制性躯体症状的鉴别度，并完成了修改后的量表信度、效度检验。本轮修改了原量表条目"4，5，29，32，39，41"，具体详见表2-1-1。

表2-1-1 《西部精神医学协会（WCPA）临床躯体症状分类量表》所修订条目与原条目对照

原条目	修改后的条目
4. 全身或肢体乏力或易疲劳	4. 迟滞症状（少言、少语、少动甚至木僵）
5. 憋气	5. 不能赋予生活的意义
29. 醒后易疲倦	29. 症状晨重暮轻
32. 感到自己的精力下降，活动减慢	32. 无价值感
39. 做事提不起兴趣	39. 做事提不起兴趣（非因精力下降）
41. 头部沉重感或紧束感	41. 肢体灌铅感

一、量表修订过程

（一）研究对象

本轮量表修订工作在四川各个研究点进行。对试点单位的入组患者使用调整后的量表测试，共纳入了测试对象 478 例，男女比例为 1∶1.4，平均年龄为（38.1±2.1）岁。

此次纳入标准为：①年龄 18～65 岁的男性和女性；②不论现有诊断，各科慢性非感染性疾病中有非单一躯体主诉的患者；③患者对躯体症状引起关注，或造成痛苦，或社会功能受到影响，三者居其一。排除标准为：①急性感染、急性创伤、围术期、慢性疾病急性发作期患者；②病情危重或临终状态；③妊娠或哺乳期女性；④物质滥用者。

（二）研究内容和方法

具体内容包括对修订条目后的《西部精神医学协会（WCPA）临床躯体症状分类量表》采用探索性因素分析和验证性因素分析的方法进行内部结构检验；并进行信度、效度指标的检测。所采用的研究工具包括 SPSS19.0，R 软件的"SEM"、SAS 软件、"proc calis"及 LISREL 专业软件。

（三）研究结果

1. 信度评估　对该量表进行了一周后重测，其重测信度如表 2-1-2 所示。

表 2-1-2　《西部精神医学协会（WCPA）临床躯体症状分类量表》修订条目后重测信度

躯体类型	α 系数	分半系数
情绪性躯体症状	0.704	0.815
抑制性躯体症状	0.613	0.652

续表

躯体类型	α 系数	分半系数
激惹性躯体症状	0.543	0.622
生物性躯体症状	0.614	0.571
想象性躯体症状	0.836	0.857
认知性躯体症状	0.691	0.650
总体	0.863	0.893

结果显示，总体上 5 个类别的检测信度良好，说明修订后的量表具有良好的稳定性。

2. 效度评估　在 2015～2016 年的现场测试入组患者中，我们对调整后的量表进行了内部结构检验。对条目调整后的分类量表进行了探索性因素分析，碎石图显示将 55 个条目聚合为 5 类信息最集中（图 2-1-1）。

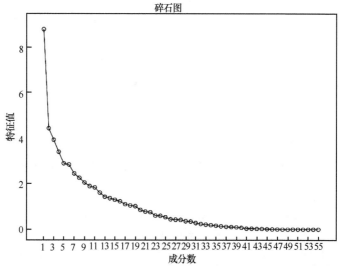

图 2-1-1　《西部精神医学协会（WCPA）临床躯体症状分类量表》
内部结构检验"碎石图"

图 2-1-1 中将 55 个条目聚合为 5 类数据信息最集中，这个结果支持本次量表修订的初衷，即将激惹性躯体症状和抑制性躯体症状加以区分，从而形成概念更为明确的躯体症状的五大心身分类。

3. 验证性因子分析　在 2015～2016 年度现场测试的入组被试中，我们对本分类量表结构进行了检验。通过对调整条目后的"量表"进行验证性因子分析，探讨数据拟合程度，其结果详见图 2-1-2。

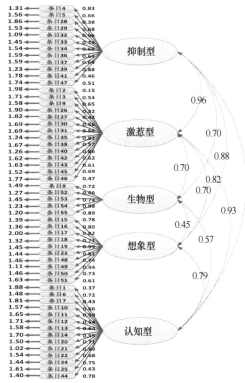

图 2-1-2　《西部精神医学协会（WCPA）临床躯体症状分类量表》
条目修订后路径图

路径图可以看出总体效度好，所有指标都满足统计学要求。尤其是抑制性躯体症状和激惹性躯体症状两者潜变量关联系数较高。

二、量表修订结果

（1）通过对《西部精神医学协会（WCPA）临床躯体症状分类量表》的修订，修改后的条目对抑制性躯体症状和激惹性躯体症状有良好的鉴别。

（2）2015～2016年度现场测试数据反映了修订后的量表内部结构性好，数据拟合度高。完成了《西部精神医学协会（WCPA）临床躯体症状分类量表（第二版）》的修订目标。

（3）关于与节律相关的症状是否成为一类独立的症状，以及"量表"是否能反映与节律问题相关症状等问题有待进一步探索和修订。

第二节　心身医学理论框架下的《西部精神医学协会（WCPA）临床躯体症状分类量表（第二版）》及其使用说明

一、量表简介

（1）有前面所描述的各方面工作，最终完成了用于临床躯体症状心身分类的《西部精神医学协会（WCPA）临床躯体症状分类量表》的修订，形成了《西部精神医学协会（WCPA）躯体症状分类量表（第二版）[WCPA Somatic Symptoms Rating Scale（second edition）]》，并完成了国家专利发明的申报（专利号：201410363067.1）。

（2）《西部精神医学协会（WCPA）临床躯体症状分类量表（第二版）》同样共55个条目，每个条目有5级评分，包括患者自评（p）和医生他评（d）两个部分。

（3）量表适应范围：本量表适用于"慢性非感染性疾病"的所有患者。

（4）"量表"适用于评估其最近4周内躯体症状的严重程度。

（5）在感染期、围术期、围产期或临终状态不适合使用该量表。

二、《西部精神医学协会（WCPA）躯体症状分类量表（第二版）》内容

（一）量表指导语

（1）请仔细阅读下面的条目，并在符合自己情况，特别是符合自己最近4周内情况的相应栏目内做上"√"符号。

（2）"量表"中的等级数字：0表示"从无"，1表示"轻度"，2表示"中度"，3表示"偏重"，4表示"严重"。

（二）量表内容

《西部精神医学协会（WCPA）临床躯体症状分类量表（第二版）》

（最近4周的症状）	0 从无	1 轻度	2 中度	3 偏重	4 严重
1. 咽喉部异物感、不适或吞咽困难；e					
2. 出现于身体任何部位的疼痛；b					
3. 感觉多汗；b					
4. 迟钝症状（少言、少语、少动）；a					
5. 不能赋予对生活的意义；a					
6. 出现肌紧张、肌肉跳动或四肢震颤等现象；e					
7. 体验到症状的性质及部位相对固定，症状清晰、生动；e					
8. 主观不适体验；c					
9. 四肢或全身发冷或发热；b					
10. 脑鸣或耳鸣；e					
11. 健忘；e					
12. 不能集中注意力；e					
13. 不能快速思考或有时脑子一片空白；e					
14. 躯体某个部位或多个部位出现"稀奇古怪"的感觉；e					

（最近4周的症状）	0 从无	1 轻度	2 中度	3 偏重	4 严重
15. 确认自己的身体出了严重问题；d					
16. 体验到的躯体不适感在身体各部分游走；d					
17. 很容易体验到躯体的各种不适；d					
18. 有许多不同种类的症状困扰您；d					
19. 如果医生告诉您"没发现您患有什么疾病"，您不能相信；d					
20. 心前区不适感；e					
21. 有短暂神志不清的感觉；e					
22. 头昏或眩晕；e					
23. 感觉躯体某部位丧失了功能；d					
24. 感觉自己缺氧；e					
25. 全身或局部肿胀感；e					
26. 入睡困难；b					
27. 睡眠浅；b					
28. 早醒；a					
29. 症状晨重暮轻；a					
30. 多梦或受梦的困扰；b					
31. 尿频；b					
32. 无动力感；a					
33. 性欲减退；a					
34. 消化不良；a					
35. 皮肤过敏；b					
36. 便秘；a					
37. 胃肠胀气；a					
38. 溃疡；b					
39. 做事提不起兴趣（非因精力下降）；a					
40. 上腹烧灼感；b					
41. 肢体灌铅感；a					

（最近4周的症状）	0 从无	1 轻度	2 中度	3 偏重	4 严重
42. 腹泻；b					
43. 恶心或呕吐；b					
44. 鼻腔异物感；e					
45. 心慌或心悸；b					
46. 一阵阵坐立不安心神不定；b					
47. 感到熟悉的东西变得陌生或不像真的（非真实感）；a					
48. 您比别人对疼痛更敏感；d					
49. 您体验到的躯体症状内容具有多样性、多变性；d					
50. 您比大多数人更担心自己的健康；d					
51. 通过公众传媒（广播、电视、报纸等）或从您认识的人那里看到、听到某种疾病后，会导致您对患这种疾病的担心，或会将自己存在的不适与之联系；d					
52. 医学实验室辅助检查；c					
53. 有明确诊断的重大疾病；c					
54. 查体发现具有诊断意义的阳性体征；c					
55. 肉眼可见的躯体损害；c					

三、量表使用说明

（一）使用举例

如所面对的患者表述具有咽喉部的不适或梗阻感，这种感觉出现频度较低，每周1～2次，而这种感觉患者已经明显地感觉到或注意到，但此项感觉不影响自身的生活，也不给本人带来明显的痛苦，对照量表的条目，此种症状符合量表的条目1喉咙异物感或吞咽困难。而该条目中对此项症状严重程度的描述包括：0级，无此症状；1级，2周内出现1～2次，基本不引起痛苦感觉；2级，1周内出现1～2次，稍微有痛苦感；3级，1周内每天出现1次，痛苦感较明显；4

级，每天出现数次，痛苦感极为明显。该患者的此项症状严重程度符合"轻度"的标准，因此记录方法如下：

（最近4周的症状）	0 从无	1 轻度	2 中度	3 偏重	4 严重
1.咽喉部异物感、不适或吞咽困难；e		√			
2.出现于身体任何部位的疼痛；b					
3.感觉多汗；b					

……

以此类推，完成 55 个条目的评分。

（二）量表评分细则

本量表采用自评/他评相结合的方式进行评估，其中条目 52、53、54、55 为临床医师评定项目，其余 51 个条目可为患者自评项目或者医生他评。逐条评分说明如下：

（1）条目 1、2、3、4、5、6、9、10、11、12、13、14、20、21、22、23、24、25、34、35、36、37、40、41、42、43、44、45、46、47 评分说明：①上述条目均包括 5 个评分等级；②0 分指无此项症状；1 分表示两周内偶尔出现（1～2 次），基本不引起痛苦感觉；2 分表示 1 周内出现 1～2 次，稍微有痛苦感；3 分表示 1 周内每天出现至少 1 次，痛苦感较明显；4 分则表示每天出现至少 1 次，痛苦感极为明显。

（2）条目 7 的评分说明：条目 7 的内容是"体验到症状的性质及部位相对固定，症状清晰、生动"。此处所说的"症状"是指任何躯体症状，如痛、痒、胀等，基于这种情况，进行如下评分：

0 分：未见症状固定、清晰。

1 分：有躯体症状，基本固定、清晰，痛苦感一般。

2 分：有躯体症状，固定、清晰，有较明显痛苦感。

3 分：有躯体症状，固定、清晰，有明显痛苦感。

4 分：有躯体症状，固定、清晰，有严重痛苦感。

（3）条目 8 的评分说明：该条目的基本内容是"主观不适体验"。

主观不适体验的内涵主要是指无明确定位的，以及无明确性质的全身性不适。该项症状的获取首先是根据患者的主述，其次，评分者根据患者描述的情况加以判断。在症状判定清楚后，根据以下条目来评分就顺理成章，该条目具体评分标准为：

0分：患者自觉无明显体验。

1分：患者安静时有轻微不适体验，活动或工作时不察觉。

2分：患者有明显不适体验，不影响正常生活及工作。

3分：患者有明显不适体验，影响正常工作及生活。

4分：医生观察到明显的痛苦的体验，作为诊断疾病的参考及依据。

（4）条目15的评分说明：条目15的具体内容为"确定自己的身体出了严重问题"。这一条目的评分需要依据两方面的信息，一是患者自己的直接表述，二是临床医师根据患者在求医行为中的具体表现，如不断要求做躯体检查，但并不相信检查所得到的阴性结果，或怀疑躯体检查所得到的结果没有自己的实际情况严重；反复不断地寻求诊疗，但对医疗措施怀疑或不认同，或不断地纠缠；患者出现"疾病先占观念"，即除了想到疾病，没法思考其他问题，同时也无法进行其他的日常活动。对这一条目的评分需在综合掌握患者信息的情况下才能准确判断。具体评分等级如下所示：

0分：不认为自己的身体有什么严重问题。

1分：虽然知道自己身体没有大的问题，但因为躯体不适而有所怀疑。

2分：比较相信自己的身体出了问题。

3分：坚信自己的身体出了较严重问题，但相信医疗可以改善。

4分：坚信自己的身体出了极严重问题，可能医疗都不能改善。

（5）条目16的评分说明：条目16的具体内容是"体验到的躯体不适感在身体各部分游走"。设置该条目的目的在于了解患者是否存在部位不固定的不适体验，至于"不适"可以包括任何负性体验，如疼痛、发冷、发热、发麻等。具体评分等级如下：

0 分：无游走性躯体不适。

1 分：躯体不适出现的部位不固定，2 周出现 1、2 次，痛苦感较轻。

2 分：躯体不适出现的部位不固定，1 周出现 1、2 次，痛苦感一般。

3 分：躯体不适在全身各处游走，每天出现 1 次，痛苦感明显。

4 分：躯体不适在全身各处游走，每天出现数次，痛苦感严重。

（6）条目 17 的评分说明：条目 17 的具体内容是"很容易体验到躯体的各种不适"。该条目有两方面含义，一是指患者很容易体验到躯体的不适，或将这种不适放大，如将睡后刚起床时很多人都可以体验到的身体沉重感做为就诊主诉；二是将一些总是容易将躯体的各种本属于正常的感受做出负性解读，如大便前的轻微腹痛、偶然感觉到的颈动脉搏动等。具体评分等级见下列标准：

0 分：对身体各部位变化不敏感，不关注。

1 分：对身体各种变化有所关注，但无痛苦感。

2 分：对身体各种变化较关注，痛苦感一般。

3 分：对身体各种变化很关注，痛苦感明显，但注意力尚可被转移。

4 分：对身体各种变化极关注，痛苦感严重，注意力无法被转移。

（7）条目 18 的评分说明：条目 18 的具体内容是"有许多不同种类的症状困扰您"。这一条目的评分主要依据受评者的主观描述，具体评分等级如下：

0 分：无症状。

1 分：有 1～2 种不同的症状存在，痛苦感较轻。

2 分：有 3 种不同的症状存在，痛苦感一般。

3 分：有 3 种以上症状存在，痛苦感明显。

4 分：有 3 种以上症状存在，痛苦感严重。

（8）条目 19 的评分说明：条目 19 的具体内容是"如果医生告诉您没发现您患有什么疾病，您不能相信"。该条目所指的"疾病"

是目前公众概念所认同的存在病理损害，即所谓"器质性疾病"，具体评分等级如下所述：

0 分：完全相信医生。

1 分：担心有器质性问题，医生告知正常后担忧念头基本打消。

2 分：虽然医生告知无器质性问题，仍有隐隐担忧，要求进一步检查。

3 分：医生告知无器质性问题，辅助检查亦正常，仍担忧是不是病没有查出来。

4 分：医生告知无器质性问题，辅助检查正常，但自己完全不相信是正常的。

（9）条目 26 的评分说明：条目 26 的具体内容是"入睡困难"。评估此项问题依据两个方面，目前国际业内对入睡困难认定的公认标准是上床后入睡时间超过 30 分钟，而本量表设定的入睡困难标准是"1 小时左右"，也就是说评定该项症状的客观标准至少大于 30 分钟，两种表述并不矛盾。此外，值得注意的是评估该项条目患者的主观体验和描述重于具体时间，即如果患者坚持认为自己存在入睡困难，那么就应该记录为有此项症状，评分等级就以出现频度，以及对本人的影响为标准，而忽略时间。

0 分：无此症状。

1 分：需要花 1 小时左右才能入睡，2 周来出现 1～2 次。

2 分：需要花 1 小时以上才能入睡，1 周出现 1～2 次。

3 分：需要花 1 小时以上才能入睡，1 周出现 3 次以上。

4 分：完全无法入眠，甚至通宵不睡，1 周来几乎天天如此。

（10）条目 27 的评分说明：条目 27 的具体内容是"睡眠浅"。睡眠浅的含义及具体评分标准如下所示：

0 分：无此症状。

1 分：睡着后感觉周围发生的事自己基本知道，但没有完全醒来。

2 分：睡着后感觉周围发生的事自己都知道，易醒，醒来可再睡去。

3 分：睡着后感觉周围的轻微声响都可将自己惊醒，醒来可再睡去。

4 分：明显睡眠感缺失，轻微响动就惊醒，且很难再睡去。

（11）条目 28 的评分说明：条目 28 的具体内容是"早醒"，其含义及具体评分标准如下所述：

0 分：无症状。

1 分：比平时早 1 小时醒来，2 周来出现 1～2 次。

2 分：比平时早 1 小时醒来，1 周出现 2 次左右。

3 分：比平时早 1 小时以上醒来，1 周出现 3 次以上。

4 分：比平时早 1 小时以上醒来，1 周来几乎天天如此。

（12）条目 29 的评分说明：条目 29 的具体内容是"症状晨重暮轻"。在此处所说的"症状"是指所有的负性体验，包括情绪及各类躯体症状。具体标准为：

0 分：无此现象。

1 分：白天负性情绪体验或各种躯体不适重于夜间，日常生活基本不影响。

2 分：白天负性情绪体验或各种躯体不适重于夜间，日常生活受到一定影响，但能够进行。

3 分：白天负性情绪体验或各种躯体不适重于夜间，日常生活不能完整进行。

4 分：白天负性情绪体验或各种躯体不适重于夜间，日常生活基本不能进行。

（13）条目 30 的评分说明：条目 30 的具体内容为"多梦或受梦的困扰"。此条目主要强调个体对梦的负性体验。睡眠研究表明，人类睡眠期间，做梦主要出现在快眼动（REM）睡眠阶段，而在成年期 REM 睡眠占总睡眠时间的 1/3～1/4，也就是说睡眠中的做梦是正常情况。有人表述自己"整夜都在做梦"，从睡眠生理角度看是不可能的，反之有人表述自己"整夜都没有梦"，从睡眠生理角度理解也是不可能的。因此，此条目主要是评价个体对梦的负性体验，如果受评者虽然回应自己有梦的体验和回忆，但没有对梦的负性体验，应视为没有此项症状。在确定患者有对梦的负性体验的情况下，可按以下标准评价该患者的程度：

0分：无症状。

1分：睡着后感觉做了好几个梦，内容较清晰，但对情绪无大的影响。

2分：睡着后感觉连着做了好几个梦，内容清晰，多为紧张恐怖的梦，醒后情绪无大影响。

3分：感觉整晚都在做梦，内容多为紧张恐怖的，醒后情绪稍受影响。

4分：感觉整晚都在做梦，内容全是紧张恐怖的，醒后紧张情绪久久不能平复。

（14）条目31的评分说明：条目31的具体内容是"尿频"。同样，这也是一项以主观体验为基础的评分，与具体次数关系不大，而与个体对该现象的体验密切相关。具体标准如下所示：

0分：无症状。

1分：自己察觉上厕所小便的次数较往常稍增多，但尚能接受。

2分：自己察觉上厕所小便的次数增多，不解则有不安的感觉。

3分：察觉自己上厕所小便的次数明显增多，解后仍有尿意，部分影响日常生活。

4分：察觉自己上厕所小便的次数明显增多，常常感觉没有解尽，严重影响日常生活。

（15）条目32的评分说明：条目32的具体内容为"无动力感"。此处的"无动力感"主要含义是"有心无力"的情况，故以"精力"作为评估该项情况的基础，而"无欲望"的情况不包括在内。

0分：无症状。

1分：感精力稍微变差，但基本不影响日常生活及工作。

2分：感精力有所下降，动作较慢，完成工作较吃力，日常生活基本能维持。

3分：感精力明显下降，动作较慢，工作难以胜任，日常生活较吃力。

4分：感精力明显下降，动作明显迟缓，完全无法工作及维持日常生活。

（16）条目33的评分说明：条目33的具体内容是"性欲减退"。具体评分等级参见下列内容。值得说明的是无论什么原因，只要出现下列情况，均应按下面的标准评分。

0分：无症状。

1分：对性生活无要求，但能配合配偶完成性行为。

2分：对性生活无要求，对配偶的性要求无法满意配合。

3分：对性生活无要求，对配偶的性要求无回应。

4分：对性生活完全无要求，尽量回避配偶的性要求。

（17）条目38的评分说明：条目38的具体内容是"溃疡"，评分标准主要以可查见的溃疡，以及对个体的影响为评定标准。

0分：无症状。

1分：两周内出现过1次口腔溃疡或胃溃疡，疼痛程度轻。

2分：1周内出现过1~2次口腔溃疡或胃溃疡，疼痛程度一般。

3分：1周内出现过数次溃疡疼痛发作，疼痛程度较重。

4分：溃疡持续存在，并经常性造成痛苦，痛苦程度重。

（18）条目39的评分说明：条目39的具体内容是"做事提不起兴趣（非因精力下降）"。该条目与条目32"无动力感"所产生的后果似乎相似，但病理心理机制则不同，如果说条目32是"有心无力"，该条目所指的则是"有力无心"或"无心无力"。即该条目强调评估的是行为的"动机"或个体的欲望，而条目32是指执行动机所具备的条件。在有的实际案例中，两者同时存在，而在有的案例中仅存在其中之一，往往是动力不足出现在前。因此在询问患者和具体评分时应注意区别。

0分：无症状。

1分：对周围事物有点提不起兴趣，但对自己以往喜欢的事物可唤起兴趣。

2分：对周围事物兴趣下降，对自己以往喜欢的事物也不如以前般感兴趣。

3分：对周围事物及自己以往喜欢的事物均明显不感兴趣。

4分：对周围事物及自己以往喜欢的事物严重提不起兴趣。

（19）条目48的评分说明：条目48的具体内容为"您比别人对疼痛更敏感"。这同样是一项要求受评者做出主观判断的问题，患者做出评价的依据是自己与周围人群的比较，同时也包含自己现在情况与自己常态状况的比较。

0分：无症状。

1分：相同受伤程度，你对疼痛的反应较别人稍显敏感。

2分：相同受伤程度，你对疼痛的反应较别人稍重，情绪反应稍明显。

3分：相同受伤程度，你对疼痛的反应较别人明显更重，情绪反应明显。

4分：相同受伤程度，你对疼痛的反应较别人明显严重，情绪反应尤其明显。

（20）条目49的评分说明：条目49的具体内容是"您体验到的躯体症状内容具有多样性、多变性"。评估的具体标准如下：

0分：症状单一固定，无多变性多样性。

1分：症状部位较多变，性质类似，造成的痛苦程度较轻。

2分：症状部位较多变，性质较多样，造成一定的痛苦。

3分：症状部位多变，性质多种多样，造成较大痛苦。

4分：症状部位多变，性质多种多样，造成严重痛苦。

（21）条目50的评分说明：条目50的具体内容是"您比大多数人更担心自己的健康"，具体含义及评分等级见下面所呈现的内容：

0分：无此情况。

1分：对身体变化较敏感，有时对自己健康有隐隐担忧。

2分：对身体变化敏感，对自己健康经常感到担忧，但注意力可被转移。

3分：对身体变化敏感，对自己健康过分担忧，需努力控制，否则注意力难以被转移。

4分：对身体变化极为敏感，对自己健康极其担忧，注意力无法转移。

（22）条目51的评分说明：条目51的具体内容是"通过公众传媒（广播、电视、报纸）或从您认识的人那里看到、听到某种疾病后，会导致您对患这种疾病的担心，或会将自己存在的不适与之联系"。具体评估标准如下：

0分：不担忧。

1分：2周来隐隐担忧，但自己能很快打消此念头。

2分：担忧出现的频率较高，1周2次左右，但自己通过查找各种资料能打消此念头。

3分：担忧频繁出现，1周3次以上或每天1次，注意力难以转移，查找资料后也难以说服自己。

4分：主动对号入座，坚信自己也身患此种疾病，担忧每天出现数次，注意力完全集中于此，无法通过各种方式打消此念头。

（23）医生借助查体或辅助检查结果所进行评估的4个条目的分别具体说明：以下每一条都是他评，具体评分是医生根据每一项描述的原则进行。

1）条目52的评分说明：条目52的具体内容是"医学实验室检查"，具体评分标准如下：

0分：所有辅助检查无阳性发现。

1分：常规检查有阳性发现，如生化常规，血常规，二便常规等。

2分：辅助检查有阳性发现，但只能作为诊断疾病的参考条件。

3分：非诊断疾病金标准的辅助检查有阳性发现，如影像学检查（MRI、CT等），心电图，肌电图，超声等，可作为诊断疾病的依据。

4分：诊断疾病的金标准所需的辅助检查有阳性发现，如病理检查，细菌培养阳性等。

（说明：辅助检查包括实验室检查、心电图、脑电图、肌电图、肺功能、X 线检查、超声检查、内镜检查、核素检查等。这些检查有上百种，每一种在疾病诊断的作用不同，可作为参考的不同评级，如同样实验室检查，有的只能作为参考，有的则作为诊断依据。每一位医生在具体疾病的判断中由以上评分项目加上医生根据辅助检查对疾病的诊断的作用来评分。）

2）条目 53 的评分说明：条目 53 的具体内容是"有明确诊断的重大疾病"，此处所指的"重大"疾病是指提示某系统或某重要器官有明显病理损害证据的疾病，如糖尿病、高血压、冠心病、甲亢、甲减等。具体评分标准如下：

0 分：目前没有明确诊断的疾病。

1 分：近 3 个月内有 1 种明确诊断的疾病。

2 分：近 3 个月内有 2 种明确诊断的疾病。

3 分：近 3 个月有 3 种明确诊断的疾病。

4 分：近 3 个月有 4 种及以上明确诊断的疾病。

3）条目 54 的评分说明：条目 54 的具体内容是"查体发现具有诊断意义的阳性体征"，具体评分标准如下：

0 分：无阳性体征。

1 分：有阳性体征，但与患者当前存在的症状或综合征不相匹配。

2 分：有阳性体征，与患者当前存在的症状或综合征部分吻合，可作为诊断疾病的提示。

3 分：有阳性体征，与患者当前存在的症状或综合征吻合，可作为诊断疾病的参考。

4 分：有明显阳性体征，与患者当前存在的症状或综合征完全吻合，可作为诊断疾病的依据。

4）条目 55 的评分说明：条目 55 的具体内容是"肉眼可见的躯体损害"，具体评分标准如下：

0 分：无肉眼可见的躯体损害。

1 分：有可见的躯体损害，但对损害部位功能不构成影响。

2分：有可见的躯体损害，对损害部位功能造成轻微影响。

3分：有可见的躯体损害，并对损害部位功能有严重影响。

4分：有可见的躯体损害，并导致损害部位功能完全丧失。

四、量表结果解读

（一）总分的意义

1. 以总分反映躯体症状的严重程度　所谓"严重程度"主要是指给患者带来的痛苦，以及对患者日常生活所带来的影响。程度越轻、总分越低；反之，程度越重，总分越高。

2. 以总分变化反映病情演变　以治疗前后量表总分的改变反映疗效，是量表总分最主要的用途之一。

3. 就具体患者而言，其疗效判断可以用总分的减分率来评估　减分率=（治疗前总分−治疗后总分）/治疗前总分。一般认为减分率≥50%为显效，≥25%为有效。

（二）单项分的意义

1. 以单项分反映具体症状的分布　症状评定量表是评定临床症状的工具，量表的单项分能反映具体临床症状类型的分布，同时也可以得到某患者哪类躯体症状最为突出的结果，而这样的结果，为制订治疗方案提供重要依据。例如，激惹性躯体症状以抗焦虑治疗为主，抑制性躯体症状以抗议于治疗为主，认知性躯体症状以非典型抗精神病药物改善认知为主等。

2. 以单项分在治疗前后的变化反映针对靶症状的治疗效果

（三）因子分析和廓图

1. 因子分的计算　因子分=组成该因子的单项评分的总和/组成该因子的项目数。

2. 以因子分析反映靶症状群的治疗结果　症状评定量表的主要

用途之一是做疗效评定,而因子分,则可反映靶症状群的治疗结果。

3. 廓图 治疗前后的廓图。廓图的意义在于了解具体患者的全面情况,为针对每个患者的个别化治疗提供依据。例如,甲、乙两个患者得分最高的因子分均为"激惹性躯体症状",但甲的次高因子分为"认知性躯体症状",而乙的次高因子分为"想象性症状",此时对甲的治疗方案应为抗焦虑药物+非典型抗精神病药物;而对乙的治疗方案应为抗焦虑药物+综合治疗(包括心理辅导、对症治疗等)。再例如,某患者被确定其躯体症状为"生物性躯体症状",表明,病理损害在负性体验的产生中起到重要作用,但正如在本共识第一章中所表达的观点一样,既然躯体症状是"不愉快主观感觉",那么任何躯体症状均应与个体的认知、情感、个性等心理因素相关,这就是为什么同样的损害在不同的个体中产生程度不同,甚至是不同形式负性体验的原因。对该类患者躯体症状的心身同治依据主要是其量表的廓图,特别是根据其次高因子分来进行。例如,某患者最高因子分提示为"生物性躯体症状",而其次高因子分提示为"激惹性躯体症状",此时,针对该患者躯体症状的治疗应该是:针对病理损害的治疗+抗焦虑治疗。

(四)因子的条目分布

四大类躯体症状分型中,情绪性躯体症状又可分为抑制性躯体症状和激惹性躯体症状两类,因此该量表可分为 5 个因子。包括:

1. 抑制性躯体症状(a) 4、5、28、29、32、33、34、36、37、39、41、47。

2. 激惹性躯体症状(b) 2、3、9、26、27、30、31、35、38、40、42、43、45、46。

3. 生物性躯体症状(c) 52、53、54、55、8。

4. 想象性躯体症状(d) 15、16、17、18、19、23、48、49、50、51。

5. 认知性躯体症状(e) 1、6、7、10、11、12、13、14、20、

21、22、24、25、44。

（五）总分及因子分计算方法

1. 因子分　因子分=该因子的各项目总和/项目数。例如，计算生物性躯体症状因子分=项目 52、53、54、55、8 的得分总和/5（5 个项目）。

2. 总分　55 个项目得分总和为症状总分。

（六）量表结果所提示意义的总结

（1）总分的意义：总分越高，表明症状越严重。

（2）因子分的意义：某因子分最高，提示了某患者所存在躯体症状的主要性质，也为治疗方案的制订提供了方向。

（3）量表廓图的意义：就像个性评定量表的作用一样，该量表的廓图可展示出患者出现躯体症状的全貌，同时也为治疗的个别化提供参考，即为治疗某患者综合治疗方案的制订提供重要参考，即为"精准治疗"提供重要参考。

（4）通过治疗前后量表的重测，通过无论是总分还是某项因子分的减分率的计算，为疗效评估及研究提供依据。

（5）量表存在条目较多，问题有待进一步准确及规范化，同时在第一章所提示的可能存在"节律性症状"的情况还未能通过测试获得相关证据等问题需在再修订时予以完善。

（曾凡敏　著）

第三章 采用心身医学理论框架下的《西部精神医学协会（WCPA）临床躯体症状分类量表（第二版）》的医学临床多中心现场测试

第一节 方 法 简 介

一、概述

基于前期研究成果，从心理测量学的角度用临床测量数据对心身医学理论下临床躯体症状分类理论假设进行了验证，并获得了心身医学视角下的临床躯体症状分类量表。同时，项目组对该理论假设进一步开展了实证研究。最后的结论是：临床躯体症状分类理论假设是成立的，临床躯体症状分类量表具有良好测量信度、效度，可作为临床躯体症状测量工具。

基于此，项目组开展了心身医学理论下的《西部精神医学协会（WCPA）临床躯体症状分类量表（第二版）》的医学临床多中心研究。在全国范围内综合医院及精神科专科医院一些科室开展了"心身医学理论框架下的躯体症状分类及诊疗的现场测试"工作。

全国 16 个学科，共计 70 个单位（以科室为单位计算）参与了此次临床试验。研究测试点单位所涉及的医学专业主要分布在神经内科、心内科、精神科、消化科、心身科、心理科、疼痛科、睡眠中心、康复科、老干科、脾胃科和男科等 16 个科室（具体信息参见表 3-1-1）。对各个参研单位进行了项目培训：使参研单位清楚了解项目的理论假设、症状分类工具、临床试验内容及操作方法。该项目连续 2 年实施现场测试。现场测试科室主要分布信息如下表。

表 3-1-1　参加《西部精神医学协会（WCPA）临床躯体症状
分类量表（第二版）》的科室

科室	比例（%）
神经内科	32.2
消化科	17.3
心身科	17.3
疼痛科	5.7
精神科	5.1
心理科	4.9
男科	3.0
心内科	3.7
睡眠中心	3.0
康复科	1.4
脾胃科	1.0
老干科	1.0
耳鼻喉科	0.4
全科	2.0
皮肤科	2.0
共计	100.0

二、现场测试流程图

本次现场测试流程图如下所示，符合纳入、排除标准的被试进行
《西部精神医学协会（WCPA）临床躯体症状分类量表》测试，根据
5 个躯体症状的亚型分别给予推荐药物方案的治疗。在基线、4 周、
12 周随访，评估被试的躯体症状严重程度及内分泌指标（图 3-1-1）。

图 3-1-1 显示，本次多中心的现场测试或研究的主要目的应该包
括：①进一步在更大的范围内验证躯体症状的分类假说；②在更大范
围内进一步验证《西部精神医学协会（WCPA）躯体症状分类量表》
的可靠性及可行性；③探索对所分类的躯体症状群治疗的有效性，从
而也从治疗的角度进一步验证躯体症状心身分类假说，并为探索有效

的治疗提供参考；④探索治疗各类躯体症状的优化治疗方案。

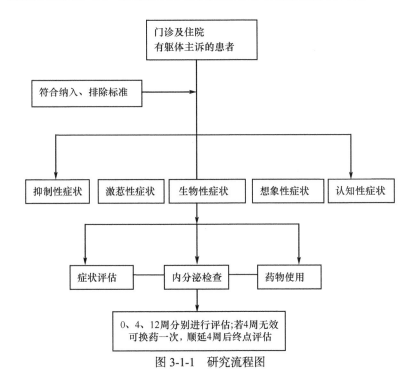

图 3-1-1　研究流程图

三、现场测试对象

（一）测试对象纳入标准

（1）年龄 18～65 岁的男性和女性；

（2）不论现有诊断，各科慢性非感染性疾病中有非单一躯体主诉的患者；

（3）患者对躯体症状引起关注，或造成痛苦，或社会功能受到影响，三者居其一。

（二）测试对象的排除标准

（1）急性感染、急性创伤、围术期、慢性病急性发作期患者；
（2）病情危重或临终不能参加本研究的患者；
（3）妊娠或哺乳期女性；
（4）物质滥用患者。

四、研究内容

（1）单次现场调查为期 12 周，共评估 3 次；生物学指标在治疗前，以及治疗后的 4、12 周共检测 3 次；所使用的心理测评工具如表 3-1-2 所示。

表 3-1-2　心理评估工具及生物学指标检测清单

症状评估	疗效评估	内分泌指标
临床躯体症状分类量表	临床疗效总评量表	HPA 轴
大五人格问卷	副反应量表	HPT 轴
		性激素
		OGTT

（2）根据量表对躯体症状的评估结果分别采用相应的药物及其他相应的方法治疗。

第二节　现场测试结果

临床躯体症状的临床治疗结果及分析

1. 入组被试基本情况　根据纳入、排除标准收集案例。截至 2016 年 6 月 15 日参研单位共回收数据 2710 例，纳入本次分析结果的有效数据为 2457 例，回收率为 90.67%。该研究的临床试验注册号为 ChiCTR-OCS-14004632。人口学资料如表 3-2-1 所示。

表 3-2-1　接受现场测试的 2457 例受试者的人口学资料

比较项目	百分比（%）
性别	
男	35.2
女	64.8
年龄	
20 岁以下	2.0
20～29 岁	8.6
30～39 岁	15.8
40～49 岁	27.7
50～59 岁	28.6
60 岁以上	17.3
受教育程度	
小学以下	6.3
小学	16.8
初中	27.3
高中或中专	23.0
大专	12.7
大学	12.2
研究生及以上	1.8
职业	
在职或学生	44.0
退休	26.1
无业或待业	28.2
婚姻状况	
未婚	7.7
同居	0.8
已婚	83.7
离异	4.6
丧偶	3.2

续表

比较项目	百分比（%）
民族	
汉族	97.8
其他少数民族	2.2
家族史	
有	8.3
无	91.7

从人口学资料中可以至少看到以下几个值得注意的特点：①躯体症状在较低文化层次人群中较为突出；②躯体症状较为集中出现在40～60 岁的人群中；③躯体症状较为集中在退休或无业人群中；④女性群体出现躯体症状高于男性。以上所提示的特点值得关注和进一步研究，特别是对"较低文化层次""女性"及"退休或无业"等特点的关注和进一步研究有助于对各类躯体症状的综合治疗。

2. 入组被试自评躯体症状对社会功能影响程度　让入组被试在症状测评中，对躯体症状对其社会功能影响程度做一评估，具体内容见表 3-2-2。

表 3-2-2　受试者自评躯体症状对社会功能影响程度

社会功能影响程度	百分比（%）
没有影响	8.5
有些影响	50.7
影响严重	40.8

在入组被试中，自评躯体症状对其社会功能有明显影响的比例为91.5%，说明躯体不适是促使患者就诊的主要原因之一。

3. 入组被试自评对躯体症状关注程度　对入组被试进行自评，考核其对躯体症状关注程度，其结果如表 3-2-3 所示。

本次现场测试共入组 2457 例，男女比例分别为 35.2% 及 64.8%；

平均年龄为（35.5±10.2）岁；入组被试的受教育程度主要集中在初
高中水平，文化水平不高；入组被试的职业状态分布情况主要以在职、
无业或待业人群居多；入组被试对躯体症状的关注程度非常高，有些
关注及非常关注程度的病例百分比为96.6%。绝大部分被试非常关注
自身的躯体症状。入组被试自评躯体症状对其社会功能影响程度百分
比为 91.5%（有些影响和影响严重两档），绝大部分被试认为躯体症
状对其社会功能影响程度大。

表 3-2-3　受试者自评对躯体症状关注程度

对躯体症状关注程度	百分比（%）
没有关注	3.3
有些关注	38.1
非常关注	58.5

4. 临床躯体症状的临床多中心测试躯体症状类型分布　统计了
临床多中心测试结果，心身医学理论框架下的临床躯体症状分类的 5
个亚型的分布情况如表 3-2-4 所示。

表 3-2-4　躯体症状类型分布

躯体症状类型	百分比（%）
抑制性躯体症状	41.9
激惹性躯体症状	21.7
想象性躯体症状	4.1
生物性躯体症状	11.2
认知性躯体症状	21.1

　　结果表明，情绪性躯体症状所占比例比较高。从 2014 年的测试
结果看，排序第一的是"激惹性躯体症状"，这比较符合实际，焦虑
是个体基本情绪的常规理念，而加上 2015～2016 年的数据以后，呈
现的结果是"抑制性躯体症状"排到了所有躯体症状的第一位，作为
现场测试的实际结果，作者表示尊重，并公开呈现，但出现这种情况

的原因可能有以下几个方面：①参与测试者"抑制性躯体症状"和"激惹性躯体症状"的识别尚未完全同意标准；②修订后的"量表"对区分两类躯体症状不够敏感和准确；③虽然根据常识，激惹性躯体症状理应多于抑制性躯体症状，但鉴于对社会功能的影响，后者就诊的群体多于前者；④当前的测试结果本来就是实际情况的真实反映。至于更准确的信息，有待于进一步的"量表"修订和现场测试。

5. 量表因素分析结果　根据医学临床多中心研究 2547 例受试者的测量数据，我们在此根据较大的多中心数据对《WCPA 躯体症状分类量表（第二版）》内部结构进行了验证，其结果如下：

（1）因素分析的适当性见表 3-2-5。

表 3-2-5　因素分析的适当性

Kaiser-Meyer-Olkin Measure of Sampling Adequacy		0.847
Bartletts Test of Sphericity	Approx. Chi-Square	6849.568
	df	1431
	Sig.	0.000

结果表明，KMO 的值大于 0.8，说明该组数据适合做因素分析。

（2）因子的累计方差贡献率见表 3-2-6。

表 3-2-6　二阶因子的累计方差贡献率

成分	总	变异（%）	累积（%）
1	7.181	39.395	39.395
2	3.479	7.217	46.612
3	3.190	6.912	53.524
4	2.163	6.895	60.419

结果表明：方差累计贡献率为 60.419，说明提取 4 个公共因子是可取的。

（3）碎石图（图 3-2-1）。

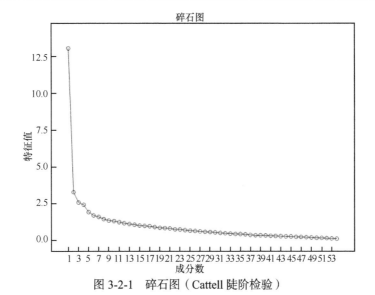

图 3-2-1　碎石图（Cattell 陡阶检验）

　　根据累计贡献率确定因子个数；以特征值是否大于等于 1 为标准；碎石检验结果共 3 个指标确定公共因素的个数为 4。现场测试数据结果再次证明了临床躯体症状分类量表的科学性，将躯体症状分为四个维度是可行的。

　　6. 治疗效果评估　根据心身医学理论下的临床躯体症状分型理论，将临床躯体症状分为 5 个亚型，并对每种躯体症状的处理给予了推荐治疗方案，具体推荐治疗方案可参看第四节。参与本项目的全国共 70 个参研点，根据推荐的治疗方案进行相应的药物治疗及心理治疗，我们将入组被试基线、1 个月后、3 个月后的躯体症状进行了评估，其结果作为治疗效果评估指标之一（表 3-2-7）。治疗效果评估包括两部分：一是躯体症状分类量表测试结果，按照国际通行原则，将躯体症状分类量表总分减分率大于或等于 25% 视为有效；躯体症状分类量表总分减分率大于或等于 50% 视为显效；二是参看内分泌检测结果的改变。

表 3-2-7　治疗前后躯体症状分类量表总分基线、4 周、12 周结果

	基线		4 周		12 周		F
	均数	标准差	均数	标准差	均数	标准差	$P<0.01$
总分	50.36	27.47	34.36	21.14	24.27	17.18	**
抑制性	51.41	27.99	35.57	21.35	24.16	16.22	**
激惹性	53.91	28.04	35.137	19.85	23.00	16.43	**
生物性	33.85	29.11	26.36	25.43	16.46	16.56	**
想象性	40.20	31.36	28.06	26.15	18.65	21.03	**
认知性	53.40	20.15	35.59	17.94	29.21	16.27	**

**提示：治疗 1 个月、3 个月后躯体症状的严重程度减轻，治疗效果明显。

　　通过分析躯体症状分类量表测评结果 1 个月、3 个月的无效、有效、显效率的构成比发现，1 个月后治疗有效所在比例最高，为 78.2%；治疗 3 个月后，显效所占比例最高，为 66.2%。内分泌指标的改变主要体现在：

　　（1）内分泌指标的改变：TSH、FT_4、TT_4、TT_3 改变明显；

　　（2）抑制性躯体症状 TT_4、FT_4 变化明显；

　　（3）激惹性躯体症状 FT_3、ACTH 改变明显；

　　（4）躯体症状整体改变显著的内分泌指标：FT_4、TT_3、TSH。

7. 临床躯体症状的人格特征分析

　　（1）量表简介：大五人格量表，即 NEO 人格量表，建立在大五人格理论的基础之上，由美国心理学家科斯塔 Costa 和麦克雷 McCrae 在 1987 年编制成，后来经过两次修订；该测验的中文版由中国科学院的心理学家张建新教授修订；属于人格理论中特质流派的人格测试工具。大五人格包括：外向性、宜人性、尽责性、情绪稳定性、开放性。

　　1）外向性：它的一端是极端外向，另一端是极端内向。外向者爱交际，表现得精力充沛、乐观、友好和自信；内向者的这些表现则不突出，但这并不等于说他们就是自我中心的和缺乏精力的，他们偏向于含蓄、自主与稳健。

2）宜人性：得高分的人乐于助人、可靠、富有同情；而得分低的人多抱有敌意，为人多疑。前者注重合作而不是竞争；后者喜欢为了自己的利益和信念而争斗。

3）尽责性：指我们如何自律、控制自己。处于维度高端的人做事有计划，有条理，并能持之以恒；居于低端的人马虎大意，容易见异思迁，不可靠。

4）情绪稳定性：得高分者比得低分者更容易因为日常生活的压力而感到心烦意乱。得低分者多表现自我调适良好，不易于出现极端反应。

5）开放性：指对经验持开放、探求态度，而不仅仅是一种人际意义上的开放。得分高者不墨守成规、独立思考；得分低者多数比较传统，喜欢熟悉的事物多过喜欢新事物。

（2）结果

1）神经质（N）：得分越低，情绪越稳定；得分越高，情绪越不稳定。将小于20.4分视为典型低分，大于38.8分为典型高分。评估结果表明，入组被试平均得分31.46分，说明躯体症状患者情绪稳定性差。

2）外倾性（E）：得分越高，性格越外向。小于26分为典型低分，大于42分为典型高分。评估结果表明：最低分为10.31分，最高分为43.1分。说明躯体症状患者有性格处于两极的特点。

3）开放性（O）：得分越高，性格越开朗。小于32分为典型低分，大于47分为典型高分。评估结果表明最低分为8.95分，最高分为29.89分。说明躯体症状患者性格不开朗。

4）宜人性（A）：得分越高，性格越随和。小于30分为典型低分，大于48分为典型高分。评估结果表明最低分为9.25分，最高分30.74分。说明躯体症状患者性格不太随和。

5）责任心（C）：得分越高，责任心越强。小于36分为典型低分，大于44分为典型高分。评估结果表明最低为11.10分，最高分为34.34分。说明躯体症状患者责任心不强。

第三节　现场测试结果的解读

　　人格是指一个人在性格、气质和能力等方面稳定的心理特征的总和，是指个体对现实事物和环境所采取的态度和习惯化了的行为。人格特征和某型性格缺陷是心身疾病易患素质的主要因素，是引发心身疾病的内因和基础。例如，性格健全者，对生活事件的易患性低，虽有较重大的生活事件，但对其心身影响不明显；性格不健全者，对生活事件的易患性高，轻度生活事件即可能导致心身疾病。本研究发现，入组的躯体症状人群中，其人格特点表现为情绪稳定性差，性格易处于两极，性格不太随和、不开朗，并且责任心不强。这些因素都是引发心身疾病的内因和基础。已有研究，Fukud 等用气质与性格问卷调查了 211 例慢性疲劳综合征患者与 90 名正常被试之间的人格差异，结果发现慢性疲劳综合征患者表现出更多的神经质倾向。

　　本研究发现，神经质的人格特质在躯体症状人群中特征显著。这一研究结果和以往研究结果取得了一致。神经质是人格特质的核心因素之一，它反映了个体感知和体验外在世界危险和混乱的程度。这一人格特质得分高的个体会报告更强烈和更频繁的负性情绪，感到不自信，经历更多的应激，以及有更多的躯体担忧。研究发现，过度夸大躯体症状也是神经质人格的基本特点之一。以躯体症状总分为因变量的研究表明，神经质人格与躯体症状间呈显著正相关。

　　临床躯体症状分类的临床多中心研究中，对不同躯体症状进行了不同的推荐方案治疗，现场测试结果提示躯体症状治疗效果显著。另一方面，我们对躯体症状的神经内分泌指标加以考察，发现 1 个月、3 个月后神经内分泌指标趋于正常的比例大大增高，与基线差异明显，达到了统计学标准（$P < 0.05$，$P < 0.01$）。结果表明，对临床症状从心身医学理论视角进行解读将其分为五个大的维度是科学、合理的。

　　在所有 2457 例入组患者中生物性躯体症状仅仅有 4.1% 的比例，这是该多中心现场测试的一个薄弱环节，很多参研点认为有了病理损

害就不再纳入病例观测组，导致在 5 个分型中生物性躯体症状入组数
量较少。根据逻辑学的充足理由律，在无法确定病理损害与躯体症状
之间存在必然联系的临床大多数情况下，对整体疾病的治疗应该包括
三个维度，即病因学治疗维度、病理生理和病理心理治疗维度，以及
症状学治疗维度。以对"心绞痛"的治疗为例，其病因应为多元化因
素，包括遗传因素、个性因素、环境因素多方面；其病理生理机制为
冠状动脉病变；其症状为激惹性躯体症状。因此其治疗理应包括：
①针对病因学方面的治疗，由于多元化的致病因素，也许对许多病例
来说，这方面的治疗很难真正完成；②病理生理治疗，即无论采用什
么方式，改善冠状动脉供血是治疗的主要目标；③对症治疗，对于此
种情况的对症治疗主要是通过强有力的抗焦虑药物的使用以减轻或
消除疼痛。"三个治疗维度"的理念是心身同治理论的具体体现，而
这种理念需要进一步验证和分享，以便得到更多临床工作者的认同。

　　通过临床多中心的现场测试数据，我们再次对《西部精神医学协
会（WCPA）临床躯体症状分类量表》进行了验证性分析，此结果再
次证明了我们在心身医学理论框架下对临床躯体症状的解读的科学
性和合理性，说明该测量工具具有良好的信度、效度，可用于临床实
践。其次在该量表提示下的临床躯体症状分类理念及实践可以为临床
躯体症状识别与治疗提供重要依据。关于治疗方案的相关解读参见第
四章。

（曾凡敏 著）

第四章 心身医学理论框架下躯体症状分类治疗的临床多中心现场测试结果总结

第一节 优化治疗方案推荐说明

一、关于优化治疗方案推荐的设想

前面已讲到，根据心身医学理念提出的躯体症状类型分为情绪性躯体症状（激惹性躯体症状和抑制性躯体症状）、认知性躯体症状、想象性躯体症状、生物性躯体症状。在第三章中，已经描述了采用WCPA躯体症状分类量表所进行的测试，分析并证实了躯体症状心身分类的存在。本章主要是描述对所分类症状的药物治疗情况。

优化治疗方案的推荐思路是根据心身医学理论对不同类型躯体症状的成分解析分别给予相应的治疗方案。例如，对于激惹性躯体症状采用抗焦虑方案治疗；对抑制性躯体症状采用用抗抑郁方案治疗；对认知性躯体症状以改善认知和调整情绪为治疗目标；对想象性躯体症状则以改善认知、调整情绪、规划生活、建立良好的人际关系，以及促进其个性成长为综合治疗目标，其中除推荐药物治疗方案外，还包括强调心理辅导对该类症状治疗的作用；对于生物性躯体症状，作者认为，既然躯体症状的实质是"不愉快的主观感觉"，以此推理，任何躯体症状均与心理因素相关。对于生物性躯体症状的分析应该是承认病理损害在产生症状中的作用，同时应排除病理损害的因素单独对个体的躯体症状进行分析从而确定对该类躯体症状的个性化治疗目标，如改善认知、调整情绪等，也就是说在针对病理损害治疗的基础上同时进行针对患者症状的心身综合治疗。

二、针对各类症状治疗的具体推荐方案

（一）治疗激惹性躯体症状的推荐方案

在前面章节已经提到本"共识"所定义的激惹性躯体症状为器官功能紊乱为基本特征的症状，如肠易激综合征、疼痛等，由于这类症状反映了器官警觉性增高的情况，因此抗焦虑治疗应该是治疗这类症状的基本原则。此外，病理性焦虑的产生源于异常的认知，因此治疗病理性焦虑应包括体验、认知及对症三个维度。基于前述考虑，对激惹性躯体症状的治疗的基本原则理应包括抗焦虑、改善认知及改善体验。根据前面的思路，激惹性躯体症状治疗的推荐方案如下：

1. SSRI 类药物（选择性 5-羟色胺再摄取抑制剂）+非典型抗精神病药物+中、长半衰期的苯二氮䓬类药物方案　本项目中针对激惹性躯体症状所推荐的 SSRI 类药物主要包括帕罗西汀、舍曲林、艾司西酞普兰和西酞普兰；基于疗效、安全性，以及临床医师，特别是非精神专科临床医师使用精神药物的习惯，本项目中所推荐的非典型抗精神病药物主要包括奥氮平和喹硫平；本项目中所推荐的中、长效苯二氮䓬类药物主要是阿普唑仑和氯硝西泮。

2. SSRI 类药物+非典型抗精神病药物+非苯二氮䓬类抗焦虑药物方案　此方案中所推荐的具体的 SSRI 类药物及非典型抗精神病药物与方案一相同，而针对那些主要以激惹性躯体症状为主诉但没有睡眠障碍的患者，此推荐方案将苯二氮䓬类药物替换成了非苯二氮䓬类抗焦虑药物。具体推荐的药物主要是坦度螺酮。在临床实践中，临床医师也可以使用此类药物中的其他药物。

3. SNRI 类药物+非典型抗精神病药物+中、长半衰期的苯二氮䓬类药物+硫必利方案　在此方案中，所推荐的具体的 SSRI 类药物、非典型抗精神病药物，以及中、长半衰期苯二氮䓬类药物均与前面相同，而推荐硫必利是特别针对疼痛症状患者。

4. 氟哌噻吨美利曲辛片+中、长半衰期苯二氮䓬类药物方案　氟哌噻吨美利曲辛片为氟哌噻吨+美利曲辛的复合制剂，前者为第一代抗精神病药物，后者为三环类抗抑郁剂，因此选择此药物的目的在于改善焦虑的体验和认知，而增加苯二氮䓬类药物是为了加强改善睡眠的效果及早期抗焦虑的效果。

5. 中成药方案　目前国内针对情绪障碍的中成药众多，研究结果不尽一致。考虑到药物的安全性，也考虑到中国患者的文化背景，以及进一步在自然临床工作环境中对中成药疗效的观察，在本次现场测试中推荐有近期研究证明对焦虑及抑郁情绪有效的乌灵胶囊和疏肝解郁胶囊作为治疗激惹性躯体症状的中成药。临床医师可以单独使用，并在较大样本的基础上对其疗效进行总结，也可以根据患者的实际情况，将上面推荐的方案作为主要治疗方案，而将这两种药物作为辅助用药。

（二）治疗抑制性躯体症状的推荐方案

本共识所指的抑制性躯体症状是器官功能抑制或弱化所表现的症状，如腹胀、厌食、功能性消化不良综合征等。同时本共识假设抑制性躯体症状是病理性抑郁情绪的躯体表现，因此抗抑郁治疗成为治疗此类症状的主要目标。此外，病理性抑郁情绪的产生首先基于歪曲的认知（不能赋予生活的意义），其次是压抑的心境，再有就是生物节律的混乱，因此对病理性抑郁的治疗应包括改善认知、改善体验及调整节律等治疗维度。同理，既然将抑制性躯体症状作为病理性抑郁治疗，在优化治疗方案的推荐中，也同样基于前面所提到的三个维度。

1. SNRI 类药物（选择性 5-羟色胺、去甲肾上腺素再摄取抑制剂）**+非典型抗精神病药物+中、长半衰期苯二氮䓬类药物方案**　由于 SNRI 类药物的双重作用，目前在精神病学界被视为主要抗抑郁剂。在该方案中所推荐的具体药物包括文拉法辛和度洛西汀，以文拉法辛为例，在 150mg 日量的情况下，其作用等同于 SSRI 类药物，即起到 5-羟色胺再摄取抑制剂的作用，当日剂量达到 225mg 或以上时，对中枢神经系统则发挥 5-羟色胺和去甲肾上腺素的双重再摄取抑制的作用，而日剂量 300mg 以上，则除了发挥 5-羟色胺和去甲肾上腺素双重再摄取抑制作用以外，还可作用于中枢神经系统的多巴胺系统。因此该类药物既可改善抑郁的感受，又可改善抑郁的认知，这便是将该类药物作为主要抗抑郁剂的原因，本共识假定抑制性躯体症状的基础是病理性抑郁，即认为抑制性躯体症状为抑郁障碍的躯体表现形式，因此将此类药物推荐为治疗抑制性躯体症状的主要药物；该方案中所推荐的具体非典型抗精神病药物仍然为奥氮平和喹硫平。之所以在推荐方案中强调使用非典型抗精神病药物，理由与对治疗激惹性躯体症状相同，即强化改善患者的认知，而对于病理性抑郁的治疗而言，改善认知显得更为重要和必要；而所推荐中、长半衰期的苯二氮䓬类药物作为该方案的组成部分之一的目的是改善患者治疗早期的感受及睡眠问题，具体药物与治疗激惹性躯体症状相同。

2. SSRI 类药物+非典型抗精神病药物+中、长半衰期苯二氮䓬类药物方案　选择非典型抗精神病药物和苯二氮䓬类药物的理由及具体推荐药物与方案一相同，此处不再赘述。此方案中所指的 SSRI 类药物主要是氟西汀。以往的研究和临床实践表明，氟西汀可作用于甲状腺轴，并改善个体的动力缺乏，由此在治疗抑制性躯体症状中推荐使用。

3. SNRI 类药物/SSRI 类药物+心境稳定剂+非典型抗精神病药物方案　在该推荐方案中选用 SNRI 类药物、SSRI 类药物及非典型抗精神病药物的理由，以及具体建议使用的药物与方案二相同。建议使用心境稳定剂的理由在于近年来精神病学界认为病理性抑郁属于节律障碍的一部分，而研究表明心境稳定剂主要治疗作用在于稳定生物节律，如情感节律。既然本共识假定抑制性躯体症状是病理性抑郁的躯体表现形式，推荐使用心境稳定剂作为治疗抑制性躯体症状的一部分就顺理成章。在此次现场测试中所推荐的心境稳定剂的具体药物包括拉莫三嗪和丙戊酸钠。碳酸锂为精神病学界公认的具有确切疗效的心境稳定剂，但考虑到药物的安全性、非精神专科临床医师对该药的熟悉程度，以及非精神科患者对该药的接受度等具体情况，故在此方案中不直接推荐，但熟悉该药的精神专科医师可根据患者的具体情况将该药纳入到治疗方案中。

4. 关于使用其他 SSRI 类药物为核心的组合方案的说明　根据以往文献报道，除氟西汀以外，其余的 SSRI 类药物均具有抗抑郁作用，因此虽然不专门推荐，在自然条件下的临床现场测试中，临床医师根据患者的实际情况采用除氟西汀以外的 SSRI 类药物，以及以此为核心的组合方案治疗抑制性躯体症状为本现场测试所接受。

5. 中成药组合方案　参见对激惹性躯体症状的治疗方案。

（三）治疗认知性躯体症状的推荐方案

关于认知性躯体症状的概念请参见第一章的相关内容。在此需要进一步说明的问题是，在临床实践中所面临的认知性躯体症状包括两个方面，一是指患者对躯体信息的负性解读，这和精神专科疑病观念的概念非常接近，而治疗的目标主要是改善患者的认知。二是符合幻觉定义的躯体症状，这类症状的特点：①符合幻觉定义，即没有客观刺激作用于感觉器官时从感觉器官直接获得的虚幻感觉；②部位相对固定；③描述清晰。而对这类情况的治疗目标包括改善认知和调整负性体验。根据前述治疗目标，对于认知性躯体症状的推荐方案包含以下情况。

1. 单独用非典型抗精神病药物方案　考虑到非精神专科医师用药习惯、对精神药物的熟悉情况，以及避免患者产生锥体外系不良反应等因素，此方案首先推荐奥氮平作为首选药物，此外临床医师也可以根据治疗目标和自己对于精神药物的用药习惯，以及用药经验选择如喹硫平或其他非典型抗精神病药物作为主要治疗药物。

2. 氟哌噻吨美利曲辛片方案　该药是一个三环类抗抑郁剂与第一代抗精神病药物的复合制剂，对认知性躯体症状推荐此药的目的是同时改善认知和不良体验。

3. 非典型抗精神病药物+SSRI 类药物方案　具体的非典型抗精神病药物仍然主要推荐奥氮平和喹硫平，而具体的 SSRI 类药物仍然推荐帕罗西汀、舍曲林、艾司西酞普兰及西酞普兰。该方案组合的目的仍然基于对认知性躯体症状的治疗目标，即改善认知和消除不良体验。

（四）治疗想象性躯体症状的推荐方案

关于想象性躯体症状概念的内涵请参见第一章。想象性躯体症状是基于暗示或自我暗示情况下所产生的一类症状。该类症状的产生比其他类症状有着更为复杂的病理生理和病理心理根源，具体地讲，这类症状的产生与个体遗产素质、早年生活的自然与人文环境、个性特征、人际关系、受教育背景、生活事件及当前的情绪状态等诸多因素相关。因此对该类症状的治疗应更为个性化，需要对治疗个体进行评估以具体确定对具体个体的当前及长久的治疗目标，所采用的药物治疗方案可根据所确定的具体治疗目标参见前面对三类症状所推荐的治疗方案进行。此外，特别值得提出的是对于这类症状的治疗，心理辅导的作用更为凸显，由于对这类症状的治疗更具个性化特征，在此不宜提出较为统一的心理干预或心理辅导模式。有关治疗这类问题的规律性的东西，特别是心理辅导方面的规律性的信息有待治疗案例的积累。

（五）治疗生物性躯体症状的推荐方案

生物性躯体症状的概念仍请参见第一章的相关内容，在此需要进一步说明的是所谓生物性躯体症状主要指的是个体存在病理损害的证据，同时又没有确切的证据表明所存在的病理损害与存在的症状之间没有必然联系的情况。本共识的基本观点是既然躯体症状是"不愉快的主观感觉"，而感觉或体验是重要的心理功能，因此任何躯体症状均与心理因素相关。基于这样的观点，对于生物性躯体症状的治疗原则是在治疗病理损害的同时，根据对患者的具体心理评估以确定对该患者的综合治疗目标，如"改善认知""调整情绪""增强心理动力"等，也就是对这类症状治疗的基本原则是"身心同治"。而关于具体推荐方案，可参见前面几类症状治疗的推荐方案。对这类症状进行自然条件下的临床现场测试目的在于希望证明任何躯体症状均与心理因素相关的理念，以及证明将躯体症状作为一个独立的治疗维度而非附属于"疾病"的必要性。

三、关于推荐方案需要说明的问题

（1）以上所有推荐方案仅仅是提示，推荐方案的提出源于文献、案例分析，以及部分临床医师的用药经验，供临床医师参考。所推荐的用药方案不限制自然条件下临床医师的用药。现场测试的结果统计以实际的临床用药信息为准。

（2）由于所推荐方案的所有药物均为上市药物，因此关于各种药相关信息如作用机制、使用剂量、不良反应，以及特殊注意事项请参考相应文献资料。原则上，本现场测试不主张违背现行原则的超剂量和违背配伍原则的用药。

（3）本着真实反应临床事件的原则，在总结临床结果时，如果绝大多数案例使用的某种药物源于一个生产厂家，则使用该药的商品名，而所使用的某种药物源于多个生产厂家则使用该药的通用名。

（4）现场测试中某治疗方案或某种药物的"排序主要反映了在治疗有效或显效的患者群体中某治疗方案或药物的使用频度，代表了当前的用药趋势"，这种排序可随着测试的深入及案例数量的增加等因素而发生变化。因此现有的排序可为目前的临床诊疗提供参考，也为临床医师提供一个进一步认识及实践的空间

（5）测试结果除为临床治疗提供重要信息以外，也是证明躯体症状心身分类假说成立证据链的一个重要环节。

第二节　躯体症状心身分类治疗结果及解读

一、心身医学理论分类框架下各类躯体症状治疗方案出现频度及分析

（一）各类躯体症状治疗结果统计

关于多中心测试研究的受试者纳入、排除标准，测试研究流程，

评估标准等信息参见第三章。在对入组患者依据《西部精神医学协会（WCPA）临床躯体症状分类量表（第二版）》进行测评后，分别参考前述的推荐方案或临床医师根据病理生理、病理心理机制所自行选定的方案进行治疗，并在治疗后 4 周、12 周分别进行随访，其目的是评估疗效、治疗方案的不良反应及其他相关情况。疗效的评估以《西部精神医学协会（WCPA）临床躯体症状分类量表（第二版）》的减分率为标准。按照临床通行标准，减分率大于或等于 25% 为有效，减分率大于或等于 50% 为显效。结果显示，使用方案 4 周和 12 周时量表总分，以及各项因子分均明显下降（$P < 0.001$）（表 4-2-1）。

表 4-2-1　躯体症状分类量表总分基线、4 周、12 周结果

项目	基线		4 周		12 周		F
	均数	标准差	均数	标准差	均数	标准差	$P < 0.001$
总分	50.36	27.47	34.36	21.14	24.27	17.18	**
抑制性躯体症状	51.41	27.99	35.57	21.35	24.16	16.22	**
激惹性躯体症状	53.91	28.04	35.13	19.85	23.00	16.43	**
生物性躯体症状	33.85	29.11	26.36	25.43	16.46	16.56	**
想象性躯体症状	40.20	31.36	28.06	26.15	18.65	21.03	**
认知性躯体症状	53.40	20.15	35.59	17.94	29.21	16.27	**

**治疗效果显著。治疗 1 个月、3 个月后，躯体症状得分显著下降。

从以上结果看，在治疗 12 周时，对各类躯体症状治疗均显著有效。统计此时各推荐方案在各类躯体症状治疗中出现的频度，并作为优化方案加以初步推广或作为完善该类症状临床治疗方案的起点是合理的。为真实反映治疗现场测试的结果，治疗方案中同时使用多个生产厂家的药物仍使用通用名，而单一使用一个生产厂家的药物则使用该厂家的商品名。此外，因为考虑到临床上单一类型症状的患者较少，一般都会是以某类型症状为主，伴有或不伴有其他类型的综合征，故在推荐方案中多使用的是联合用药，这样会使得不同类型的症状均得到缓解；然而不可避免的是，药物的联合必然增添了副反应的发生

频率, 这需要临床医师综合判断利弊做出方案选择。故为了临床实用需要, 我们在总结方案时分别总结了每项躯体类型的单一用药频度排序, 以及联合方案用药频度排序。

(二) 对激惹性躯体症状的治疗

从表 4-2-1 和表 4-2-2 中可以看到, 在现场测试中治疗激惹性躯体症状 12 周时单药方案主要以 SSRI 类药物、希德 (坦度螺酮) 及 SNRI 类药物为主, 在复合方案中黛力新 (氟哌噻吨美利曲辛片) 使用频率最高, 然后是以 SSRI 或 SNRI 类药物为核心的方案, 并在此基础上或合并苯二氮䓬类药物 (以长半衰期的氯硝西泮为主) 或合并非典型抗精神病药物 (奥氮平或喹硫平出现频率最高) 或合并另一种改善情绪的药物 (以希德、舒肝解郁胶囊、乌灵胶囊出现频率最高)。现场测试结果与我们的推荐思路及方案相符合, 且推荐方案中具体药物的治疗剂量均为临床常用的治疗剂量。关于治疗方案及所使用药物频度的排序请见表 4-2-2, 表 4-2-3, 关于所使用药物的日剂量参见表 4-2-4。

表 4-2-2　治疗激惹性躯体症状单药方案排序

使用频度顺序	用药方案
1	SSRIs 类药物[具体药物依次为盐酸帕罗西汀、艾司西酞普兰 (来士普)、西酞普兰 (喜普妙)、盐酸舍曲林 (舍曲林)]
2	坦度螺酮 (希德)
3	SNRI 类药物[依次为度洛西汀 (欣百达)、文拉法辛 (博乐欣)]
4	奥氮平 (再普乐)
5	舒肝解郁胶囊

表 4-2-3　治疗激惹性躯体症状联合用药方案排序

使用频度顺序	用药方案
1	氟哌噻吨美利曲辛片
2	SSRI 类药物+氯硝西泮 (其中 SSRI 类药物具体使用频度依次为艾司西酞普兰、盐酸帕罗西汀、舍曲林、西酞普兰)
3	SNRI 类药物+苯二氮䓬药物 (SNRI 类药物具体使用频度依次为文拉法辛、度洛西汀; 苯二氮䓬类药物的具体使用频率依次为氯硝西泮、阿普唑仑)

续表

使用频度顺序	用药方案
4	SSRI 类药物（具体使用频率依次为舍曲林、艾司西酞普兰、盐酸帕罗西汀）+坦度螺酮+非典型抗精神病药物（具体使用频率依次为奥氮平、喹硫平）
5	SSRI 类药物[具体使用频率依次为艾司西酞普兰、盐酸氟西汀（百忧解）、舍曲林]+奥氮平
6	SSRI 类药物（舍曲林、盐酸帕罗西汀）+舒肝解郁胶囊
7	SSRI 类药物（舍曲林、盐酸帕罗西汀）+乌灵胶囊

表 4-2-4　治疗激惹性躯体症状用药方案中药物日剂量范围

药物名称	剂量范围	序号药物名称	剂量范围
盐酸帕罗西汀	20～50mg	氟哌噻吨美利曲辛片	1～3 片
艾司西酞普兰	5～20mg	文拉法辛	75～225mg
盐酸氟西汀	20～40mg	奥氮平	2.5～10mg
度洛西汀	60～120mg	喹硫平	50～100mg
舍曲林	100～150mg	坦度螺酮	15～45mg
西酞普兰	20～40mg	舒肝解郁胶囊	720～1440mg
氯硝西泮	1～3mg	阿普唑仑	0.4～1.2mg
乌灵胶囊	3～9 片		

（三）对抑制性躯体症状的治疗

12 周治疗方案频度排序及方案中药物剂量范围见表 4-2-5～表 4-2-7。其中显示现场测试中抑制性躯体症状 12 周时单药方案主要以 SSRI 类药物、坦度螺酮，以及 SNRI 类药物使用频率最高；而复合方案使用频度则是依次以氟哌噻吨美利曲辛片、SSRI 类药物和 SNRI 类药物为核心所组合的方案。在治疗抑制性躯体症状中，治疗方案出现的频度及具体用药与治疗激惹性躯体症状方案及具体用药相似，分析其原因主要有以下几个方面：①以往的相关研究显示出现频度高的方案中所使用的各类药物兼有抗抑郁和抗焦虑两方面的作用，而对病理性焦虑、抑郁两方面作用更为精准的优化治疗方案的产生有待于治疗案例的继续积累；②根据心理学的基本原理，以及对异常情绪发展过程的思考，焦虑情绪应该首先被视为基本情绪，与正常的生理与心理过程密切相关。情绪障碍的发生以应激为起点（包括生理应激和心理应激），在"应激"的作用下，个体产生焦虑。在此所说的焦虑包括心理应激含义下的焦虑和躯体应激层面意义上的焦虑。前者可出现像精神疾病分类目录中所描述的创伤后应激障碍、广泛性焦虑、惊恐障碍、社交焦虑障碍、强迫障碍、睡眠障碍等方面的表现，后者则可表现出血压改变、糖代谢异常、内分泌功能异常、激惹性消化系统症状、疼痛等情况。在应激不能消除，或在应激基础上产生"次级应激源"从而使个体出现连续应对应激的情况（如患肿瘤个体在患肿瘤以后造成失业、家庭关系危机、家庭经济状况窘迫等情况），或由于个体个性缺陷造成应对危机不当等情况下个体的焦虑状态就可能或作为体验或作为躯体形式长期存在。而病理性焦虑长期存在的结果可以出现两种情况，一是出现焦虑的衰竭，此时个体可表现为动力缺乏、兴趣下降、情绪低落等，当个体处于持续应激状态下，HPA轴的活性过度，皮质醇增高可以导致中枢神经系统某些结构如海马、杏仁核前额叶皮质的损害，导致认知功能异常，从而发生病理性抑郁，而体现在躯体方面，则出现抑制性躯体症状。从以上各方面研究进行的推论可看出，焦虑和抑郁之间有着千丝万缕的联系，难以截然分开，这也应该是激惹性躯体症状和抑制性躯体症状在治疗方面治疗方案较为相似的原因之一。同样，关于治疗两类症状更为精准的优化治疗方案的产生有赖于临床治疗案例的积累、分析和观察。此外，根据以上焦虑、抑郁发展的连续过程的分析，临床诊断中对患者实际处于何种状态的判断比给其贴上一个诊断名词的"标签"更有实际意义。当然得到更为精准的优化治疗方案的前提是躯体症状分类量表工具的继续优化。

表 4-2-5　治疗抑制性躯体症状单药方案出现频度排序

出现频度排序	治疗方案
1	SSRI 类药物（具体药物使用频度依次为盐酸帕罗西汀、艾司西酞普兰、西酞普兰、舍曲林、盐酸氟西汀）
2	坦度螺酮

续表

出现频度排序	治疗方案
3	SNRI 类药物（具体药物使用频度依次为度洛西汀、文拉法辛）
4	奥氮平
5	舒肝解郁胶囊
6	乌灵胶囊

表 4-2-6　治疗抑制性躯体症状联合用药方案出现频度排序

出现频度排序	治疗方案
1	氟哌噻吨美利曲辛片
2	SNRI 类药物＋苯二氮䓬类药物（SNRI 类药物具体用药频度依次为文拉法辛、度洛西汀）；苯二氮䓬类药物具体药物的使用频度依次为阿普唑仑、氯硝西泮）
3	SSRI 类药物＋苯二氮䓬类药物（SSRI 类药物具体用药频度依次为艾司西酞普兰、盐酸氟西汀、盐酸帕罗西汀、舍曲林、西酞普兰）
4	SNRI 类药物＋奥氮平＋苯二氮䓬类药物（其中 SNRI 类药物具体药物具体使用频度依次为度洛西汀、文拉法辛）
5	SSRI 类药物＋奥氮平（其中 SSRI 类药物具体药物使用频度依次为艾司西酞普兰、盐酸氟西汀、舍曲林）
6	SSRI 类药物＋中成药（SSRI 类药物具体药物使用频度依次为舍曲林、盐酸帕罗西汀；而中成药为舒肝解郁胶囊、乌灵胶囊）

表 4-2-7　抑制性躯体症状用药方案中药物的日剂量

药物名称	日剂量范围	药物名称	日剂量范围
氟哌噻吨美利曲辛片	1～3 片	文拉法辛	75～225mg
盐酸帕罗西汀	20～60mg	坦度螺酮	10～60mg
舍曲林	50～150mg	奥氮平	2.5～15mg
艾司西酞普兰	10～20mg	喹硫平	50～100mg
西酞普兰	15～40mg	氯硝西泮	1.5mg
盐酸氟西汀	20～40mg	乌灵胶囊	3～9 片
度洛西汀	60～120mg	舒肝解郁胶囊	720～1440mg

（四）对认知性躯体症状的治疗

12 周治疗方案频度排序及方案中药物剂量范围见表 4-2-8～表 4-2-10。现场测试中对认知性躯体症状治疗 12 周时单药方案用药频率排序最高的依次为 SSRI 类药物、坦度螺酮和度洛西汀，其次是奥氮平。关于认知性躯体症状正如本章第一节已经描述过的那样，此处所指的认知性躯体症状包括两个方面的含义，一是对躯体各种感受的负性解读，二是指符合幻觉特征的躯体症状。前述两种情况均与个体的认知功能异常密切相关，因此治疗应该以改善认知功能为主，同时辅以改善负性情绪，以促进其症状消失。测试用药频度及药物种类的选择基本符合这一治疗理念。只是在使用药物排序中抗焦虑剂的使用频度似乎高于改善认知功能的非典型抗精神病药物。这种结果提示：①符合调整情绪是改善认知功能的重要环节，关于这一观点请参见第一章，特别是参见对认知层面焦虑的描述；②由于此处所统计的药物使用频度是基于治疗 12 周后对有效案例的统计，因此有必要反思分类量表的准确性，即在以后的现场测试中应进一步注意对情绪性症状和认知性症状的区别；③从心理学角度理解，认知过程、情感过程及意志过程是三个相互关联不能够截然分开的过程，在治疗认知性躯体症状中调整负性情绪的药物与改善认知的药物联合使用以取得更好的效果就顺理成章，只是需要进一步积累治疗案例以便更准确地体现对此类症状的优化治疗。

表 4-2-8　治疗认知性躯体症状单药方案出现频度排序

出现频度排序	用药方案
1	SSRI 类药物（具体用药排序依次为艾司西酞普兰、舍曲林）
2	坦度螺酮
3	度洛西汀
4	奥氮平

表 4-2-9　治疗认知性躯体症状联合用药方案出现频度排序

出现频度排序	用药方案
1	氟哌噻吨美利曲辛片
2	SSRI 类药物+坦度螺酮+非典型抗精神病药物（SSRI 类药物具体用药排序依次为舍曲林、艾司西酞普兰、盐酸帕罗西汀；非典型抗精神病药物具体用药依次为奥氮平、喹硫平）

续表

出现频度排序	用药方案
3	坦度螺酮＋苯二氮䓬类药物（苯二氮䓬类药物具体的用药依次为劳拉西泮、阿普唑仑）
4	SNRI 类药物＋坦度螺酮＋奥氮平（SNRI 类药物具体用药排序为度洛西汀、文拉法辛）
5	SSRI 类药物＋非典型抗精神病药物＋苯二氮䓬类药物（SSRI 类药物具体用药排序依次为艾司西酞普兰、盐酸帕罗西汀、舍曲林；非典型抗精神病药物的具体使用依次为奥氮平、喹硫平；苯二氮䓬类药物的具体用药为：劳拉西泮、阿普唑仑）
6 （本栏目内的两个方案在实际测试中出现频度相同）	①SSRI 类药物＋奥氮平（此方案中使用的 SSRI 类药物依次为艾司西酞普兰、帕罗西汀） ②度洛西汀＋坦度螺酮＋苯二氮䓬类药物（苯二氮䓬类药物的具体用药为劳拉西泮、阿普唑仑）
7	帕罗西汀＋舒肝解郁胶囊

表 4-2-10　认知性躯体症状用药日剂量

药物名称	日剂量范围	药物名称	日剂量范围
舍曲林	50～150mg	奥氮平	1.25～10mg
文拉法辛	75～150mg	喹硫平	50mg
度洛西汀	60～120mg	劳拉西泮	0.5mg qn
西酞普兰	5～20mg	阿普唑仑	0.2～0.8mg qn
盐酸帕罗西汀	10～40mg	舒肝解郁胶囊	720～1440mg qd
氟哌噻吨美利曲辛片	0.5～3 片		
艾司西酞普兰	10～20mg		
坦度螺酮	10～30mg		

（五）对想象性躯体症状的治疗

对想象性躯体症状治疗 12 周后治疗方案频度排序及方案中药物剂量范围见表 4-2-11～表 4-2-13。统计结果显示现场测试中治疗想象性躯体症状 12 周时，有效病例的单药方案几乎全部以 SSRI 类药物、SNRI 类药物、乌灵胶囊、舒肝解郁胶囊等改善情绪方面的药物为主；合并用药方案也基本呈现这种趋势。正如第一章所描述的那样，想象性躯体症状基于暗示、自我暗示产生，暗示是在一定的环境下和在一定的情绪气氛中，个体对来自外界的影响无条件接受的情况。个体暗示性最高的年龄段是 5～7 岁，或者笼统地讲，应该在青春前期，成为个体个性发育不成熟的一部分。到成年期随着个性的成熟暗示性降低，而如果在成年期还保持着未成年期的高暗示性，这就形成了发生想象性躯体症状的人格基础。因此，治疗想象性躯体症状的基本目标有两个方面：一是降低其暗示性，二是改善其认知功能。抗焦虑药物可以降低个体的警觉性，因而可以降低其暗示性，而非典型抗精神病药物则可改善认知功能，这便是在现场测试中这两类药物使用频度高，且多个测试单位用药方向较为一致的原因。至于是否以抗焦虑药物为主而辅以非典型抗精神病药物就是治疗想象性躯体症状的最佳治疗有待于治疗案例的继续积累。同时值得再次一提的是，根据想象性躯体症状产生的病理心理基础，对该类症状的治疗除药物治疗以外，心理辅导应该是重要的治疗环节。对于这方面的问题也有待于治疗案例的继续积累。

表 4-2-11　治疗想象性躯体症状单药方案出现频度排序

用药频度排序	用药方案
1	SSRI 类药物（具体药物使用频度依次为艾司西酞普兰、舍曲林、西酞普兰）
2	SNRI 类药物（具体药物使用排序依次为度洛西汀、文拉法辛）
3	乌灵胶囊
4	舒肝解郁胶囊

表 4-2-12　治疗想象性躯体症状合并用药方案出现频度排序

用药频度排序	合用药方案
1	氟哌噻吨美利曲辛片
2	SSRI 类药物+坦度螺酮＋非典型抗精神病药物[SSRI 类药物具体药物使用频度依次为舍曲林、盐酸帕罗西汀、艾司西酞普兰；非典型抗精神病药物具体用药频度依次为奥氮平、喹硫平、阿立哌唑（博思清）]
3	坦度螺酮＋苯二氮䓬类药物（具体用药依次为劳拉西泮、阿普唑仑）

续表

用药频度排序	合用药方案
4 （同一栏目内所列的两个方案出现频度相同）	SNRI 类药物＋苯二氮䓬类药物（SNRI 类药物具体用药依次为度洛西汀、文拉法辛；苯二氮䓬类药物具体用药依次为劳拉西泮、阿普唑仑） SSRI 类药物＋苯二氮䓬类药物（SSRI 类药物具体用药依次为盐酸帕罗西汀、西酞普兰、艾司西酞普兰；苯二氮䓬类药物具体用药依次为劳拉西泮、阿普唑仑）
5	SNRI 类药物＋非典型抗精神病药物＋苯二氮䓬类药物（此方案中 SNRI 类药物的具体用药主要是度洛西汀；非典型抗精神病药物依次为喹硫平、奥氮平；苯二氮䓬类药物依次为劳拉西泮、阿普唑仑）

表 4-2-13　治疗想象性躯体症状使用药物的日剂量

药物名称	日剂量范围	药物名称	日剂量范围
舍曲林	100～150mg	喹硫平	12.5～50mg
盐酸帕罗西汀	30～50mg	奥氮平	2.5～10mg
度洛西汀	30～60mg	阿立哌唑	5～10mg
艾司西酞普兰	5～20mg	氟哌噻吨美利曲辛片	1～2 片
西酞普兰	20～40mg	舒肝解郁胶囊	720～1440mg
文拉法辛	75～225mg	乌灵胶囊	3～9 片
奥氮平	2.5～7.5mg qn	劳拉西泮	0.5～1.5mg
坦度螺酮	20～60mg qd	阿普唑仑	0.2～0.8mg qn

（六）对生物性躯体症状的治疗

　　12 周治疗方案频度排序及方案中药物剂量范围见表 4-2-14～表 4-2-16。结果显示现场测试中生物性躯体症状 12 周时单药方案几乎全部以 SSRI 类药物、SNRI 类药物、氟哌噻吨美利曲辛片、苯二氮䓬类药物，以及舒肝解郁胶囊、乌灵胶囊等具有抗焦虑作用的药物为主。这与第一章所表述的"生物性躯体症状"的含义相符合，承认病理损害在这类症状中的作用，同时强调个体认知、情绪、个性乃至现实生活状况对产生症状或对症状严重程度的影响。因此，对生物性躯体症状的治疗应该包括两个部分，一是对病理损害的治疗，二是评估患者的心理状态并给予相应的治疗。从生物学角度看，负性体验的产生机制与中枢神经系统上行系统的被激活和下行系统的脱抑制直接相关，而上行系统是否被激活和下行系统是否脱抑制与心理因素关系密切，特别是与情绪因素关系密切。例如，在激烈的战争氛围中，由于参战个体处于高度应激的激情状态下，对所产生的损伤，甚至较为严重的损伤都可毫无察觉就是最好的例证。因此，在本次测试中使用抗焦虑药物降低个体的警觉水平，使由病理损害所产生的负性体验减轻甚至消除就顺理成章。那么，对此类症状所使用的药物同时也有抗抑郁功能，减轻躯体症状是否也与抗抑郁作用相关呢？这种判断不太可能成立，因为抑郁的病理心理过程是导致个体警觉性下降，从而使其对来自自身或外界损伤的敏感性下降，在此状态下自然负性体验程度也会下降，病理性抑郁的极端状态是"抑郁性木僵"，此时个体对来自外界的刺激或较为严重的损伤基本没有生理或心理反应。根据现场测试的结果，至少目前可以得到的结论是治疗生物性躯体症状的心身同治的基本原则是在对病理性损害治疗的基础上联合使用某类抗焦虑药物。至于治疗生物性躯体症状更为精准地使用抗焦虑药物、是否对有的患者也需要重点改善认知，以及是否对有的患者使用镇静-催眠药物或是否还可配合使用心理辅导等问题，有待治疗案例进一步积累。此外，为真实反映临床事件，临床测试中发现治疗生物性躯体症状存在"SSRI 类药物 + 氟哌噻吨美利曲辛片"的治疗方案，统计发现，该方案的使用频度较高，而且有效。但氟哌噻吨美利曲辛片含有三环类抗抑郁剂成分和典型抗精神病药物成分，是一个联合制剂，本来就具有抗焦虑作用，同时也具有改善认知的作用，再合并使用SSRI 类药物似乎没有必要，同时三环类药物合并 SSRI 类药物有增加不良反应的风险。鉴于前述原因，该治疗方案不宜作为今后临床实践中治疗生物性躯体症状或治疗其他类躯体症状的推荐方案，因此也没有在排序表中列出。

表 4-2-14　治疗生物性躯体症状单药治疗方案出现频度排序

出现频度排序	用药方案
1	SSRI 类药物（具体用药频度依次为舍曲林、艾司西酞普兰、盐酸帕罗西汀）、西酞普兰）
2	SNRI 类药物（具体用药频度依次为度洛西汀、文拉法辛）
3	舒肝解郁胶囊
4	乌灵胶囊

表 4-2-15　治疗生物性躯体症状联合用药方案出现频度排序

出现频度排序	用药方案
1	氟哌噻吨美利曲辛片
2	度洛西汀＋奥氮平＋氯硝西泮
3	舍曲林＋苯二氮䓬类药物（具体用药频度依次为氯硝西泮、阿普唑仑、劳拉西泮）

表 4-2-16　治疗生物性躯体症状具体用药的日剂量

药物名称	日剂量范围	药物名称	日剂量范围
舍曲林	50～150mg	氟哌噻吨美利曲辛片	1～2 片
文拉法辛	75～225mg	坦度螺酮	10mg
西酞普兰	20～60mg	阿普唑仑	0.2～0.4mg
盐酸帕罗西汀	20～60mg	劳拉西泮	0.5～1mg
艾司西酞普兰	15～20mg	氯硝西泮	1～2mg
舒肝解郁胶囊	1440mg	乌灵胶囊	3～9 片

二、推荐方案中不良反应排序

　　治疗第 4 周以后，报告的不良反应排序依次为口干、便秘、嗜睡、肌肉强直，12 周后不良反应排序为便秘、口干、体重增加、头痛。在临床观察中没有发现以上所描述的不良反应达到影响个体社会功能或产生危及健康的状况，因此总的来说，推荐方案被证明是安全的。此外，选择什么样的治疗方案有待临床医师对具体患者及治疗目标的综合评估。

三、对现场测试结果需要说明的问题

（1）根据治疗效果，以及在较为大宗的案例治疗中的出现频度，以上各推荐方案可以作为优化方案用于临床治疗中。但所有推荐方案为此次参与定制共识的团队制订和采用，可能存在认识的局限性及临床经验的局限性，因此目前的"优化治疗方案"仅代表 2014～2016 年的结果，而在更大范围内的临床实践及治疗方案的进一步优化很有必要。

（2）在情绪性躯体症状及认知性躯体症状的所有方案中，出现以丙戊酸钠缓释片、丙戊酸镁缓释片、拉莫三嗪为主的单药方案及其与其他药物的联合方案，并且治疗结果有效。由于这类药物不在推荐方案范围以内，同时出现频度较低，在此没有在相应的排序表中列出。但这是一个值得注意的趋势，因为这类药物属于心境稳定剂，最近几年的研究资料表明，这类药物具有稳定生物节律的作用，心境稳定仅仅是其功能的一个方面。因此将来的工作是应该继续注意积累采用心境稳定剂治疗的案例，探索是否存在"节律性躯体症状"的可能。

（孙学礼　曾凡敏 著）

第三节　各类躯体症状治疗的案例

一、以疼痛为主要表现的认知性躯体症状案例

患者刘某，男性，35 岁，已婚。左前臂针刺感 2 年。患者 2 年前因车祸致左上肢前臂轻微划伤，皮肤红肿，未出血，伴疼痛，自行乙醇消毒后红肿消退，疼痛减轻。但患者半个月后逐渐发现，每当左前臂接触衣物之后就产生针刺感，犹如一根根细针排列整齐并密集扎在皮肤上，伴轻微疼痛，感觉为持续性，脱离衣物后针刺感消失，疼痛缓解；后来发现接触其他物体也有此现象。患者症状较轻，疼痛可

忍受，不影响睡眠，但严重影响患者情绪，给患者工作及生活带来困扰，于多家医院反复就诊。查体：左上肢无畸形无包块，皮肤无红肿热痛，肌力、肌张力正常，活动正常。辅助检查：X线检查、双上肢和颈部磁共振及神经电生理检查均未见异常。诊断"疼痛待诊"。先后使用局部止痛药酮洛芬及口服药物阿司匹林、布洛芬等治疗，同时辅助物理治疗光疗法及温热疗法，均可不同程度减轻疼痛感，但针刺感仍持续存在。考虑患者症状与认知因素相关，给以服用奥氮平10mg/d，2周后针刺感减轻，疼痛消失，3周后完全好转。

治疗者体会：从症状分析，患者左前臂针刺感是受伤后出现的，容易认为是因为损伤引起的慢性疼痛。查体及辅助检查均未见异常，用止痛药无明显缓解，不考虑炎性或神经病理性疼痛可能。结合患者症状性质特征：①针刺感符合幻觉的特征，即在没有针刺的情况下产生针刺感；②体验的性质及部位固定；③症状描述清晰；④无明显病理生理性因素。考虑是认知过程问题导致了躯体不适感。所以，治疗应从改善患者对症状的认知，改变患者体验角度出发。从治疗结果来看，用多种止痛药及物理治疗均无明显效果，而改善认知的药物奥氮平则效果显著，故考虑认知性躯体症状的可能性。

二、以幻觉为特征的认知性躯体症状案例

患者王某，男性，40岁，已婚。右脚踩鹅卵石感4年。患者4年前无明显诱因出现右脚踩鹅卵石感，行走于平坦的地面时便感觉踩踏于尖锐的鹅卵石上，伴疼痛，脚离开地面时此症状消失。该症状导致患者跛行，疼痛虽可忍受，但严重影响患者情绪，给患者工作及生活带来困扰，于多家医院反复就诊。查体：双下肢无畸形、无包块，皮肤无红肿热痛，肌力、肌张力正常，活动正常。辅助检查包括X线检查、双下肢磁共振及神经电生理检查均未见异常。诊断"右脚感觉异常待诊"。先后使用局部止痛药法斯通及口服药物阿司匹林等治疗，同时辅助光疗法及温热疗法，均无明显效果。因患者疼痛，考虑患者为激惹性症状，给以丁螺环酮30mg/d抗焦虑治疗，患者症状未

见明显改善。1个月后重新分析患者的症状，踩鹅卵石感符合幻觉特征，故按照幻觉来处理，给以服用奥氮平 15mg/d，两周后踩鹅卵石感变为踩细沙感，疼痛消失，五周后完全好转。

治疗者体会：从症状分析，患者主观体验踩鹅卵石感为主要症状而附带疼痛。但临床诊疗中容易误认为疼痛为主要症状而忽视主观体验踩鹅卵石感。查体及辅助检查均未见异常，用止痛药及抗焦虑药无明显缓解，不考虑炎性或神经病理性及焦虑引起的疼痛可能。结合患者症状性质特征：①踩鹅卵石感符合幻觉的特点，即没有在踩鹅卵石的情况下产生了踩鹅卵石感；②体验的性质及部位固定；③症状描述清晰；④无明显病理生理性因素。考虑是认知障碍导致了躯体不适感。所以，治疗应从改善患者对症状的认知，改变患者体验角度出发。从治疗效果来看，按照幻觉来处理效果显著，故考虑认知性躯体症状可能。

三、以异常感觉为特征的认知性躯体症状案例

患者李某，女性，39 岁，已婚，无业。主诉"头里有长条状物不断搅动 6 月余，情绪焦虑抑郁 3 个月"。患者诉 6 个月前无明显诱因渐渐出现头晕头胀感觉，感颅内有长条状物体不断搅动，体位变动时加重，体验清晰生动，位置较固定。伴有胸闷、气短，伴有心慌、阵发性坐立不安，伴有恶心，伴有睡眠差，主要为入睡困难，易醒。于当地医院神经内科就诊，经神经系统查体及头颅 MRI 检查提示"未见明显器质性病变"，给予营养神经扩血管药物治疗，病情未见明显好转。患者对于医生告知的"未见明显器质性病变"不相信，3 个月前伴随出现焦虑抑郁情绪，兴趣下降，担心、担忧自己的躯体症状，遂入华西医院精神科门诊就医，诊断为"躯体形式障碍"，给予临床躯体症状分类量表首次评估，结果为：激惹性躯体症状因子分 1.50，抑制性躯体症状因子分 1.50，想象性躯体症状因子分 1.40，生物性躯体症状因子分 0.80，认知性躯体症状因子分 1.40。查甲状腺功能、皮质醇、促肾上腺皮质激素、性激素、糖耐量试验均在正常范围。按情绪性躯体症状给予度洛西汀 60～90mg/d，奥氮平 2.5～5mg/d，氯硝

西泮 1～3mg/d 等治疗。1 个月后患者对疾病的焦虑抑郁情绪明显缓解，心慌、气短及睡眠差等症状完全消失，但仍诉颅内有条状物体搅动，且严重时搅动物体会断裂并发出刺耳金属声音。再次复评临床躯体症状分类量表，结果为：激惹性躯体症状因子分 0.36，抑制性躯体症状因子分 0.67，想象性躯体症状因子分 0.21，生物性躯体症状因子分 0，认知性躯体症状因子分 1.20。因认知因子突出，在原配伍药物基础上，加大奥氮平用量至 10mg/d 继续治疗。治疗 2 个月后患者自述焦虑抑郁情绪完全消失，颅内物体搅动感觉少了，减少了 70%。目前尚未治疗满 3 个月。

治疗体会：患者以躯体症状首发，主要表现为感颅内有长条状物体不断搅动、断裂并发出刺耳金属声音，因症状久治未愈，伴随出现较为严重的焦虑抑郁情绪，故首次就诊，临床躯体症状分类量表评估结果以情绪性因子突出，此时易误诊为情绪障碍为主的精神疾病而单用抗焦虑抑郁药物，但考虑到躯体症状病程更长，且情绪为伴发症状，故按躯体形式障碍治疗，给予 SNRI 类药物对抗躯体症状及焦虑抑郁情绪+小剂量非典型抗精神病药物改善认知并从而缓解焦虑及改善睡眠。治疗后情绪症状明显缓解，转而突出其主要问题，评估为认知性躯体症状，症状性质被描述为生动且位置相对固定，加大非典型抗精神病药物改善认知，疗效良好。临床患者症状往往复杂而非单一，此例患者提示我们，不同分类的症状之间可能以某种因子为主但并不排斥共存，治疗不应只局限于主要因子症状或临床诊断针对治疗，而是以量表的客观评判结果对相应因子症状给予针对性强的药物种类及剂量，这样可能会取得更好的临床疗效。

四、激惹性+认知性躯体症状案例

患者马某，男性，31 岁，工人。因"阵发性手脚麻木 7 年，肌肉跳动感 5 年"前来就诊。患者 7 年前逐渐出现感手脚部多处发麻，每次持续数分钟，2～3 次每月。5 年前上述症状逐渐加重，手部发麻时不能拿物品，并出现阵发性肌肉跳动感。患者述手臂、背部及下肢均有肌肉跳动的感觉,起初每月只有几次,天气变化时发作更为频繁。半年前上述症状加重,手脚发麻时出现酸胀感,肌肉跳动感平均每天发作 3～4 次。病程中多梦,睡眠浅。患者自述梦很多,睡觉时常常因为手脚发麻而醒来,白天没有精神,经常心慌,坐立不安。患者对症状非常关注,觉得自己得了大病,四处求医。反复就诊于神经内科、神经外科、中医科,多次行肌肉电生理检查、胸椎 X 线、腰椎 X 线、颈椎胸椎 MRI、头颅 CT 等辅助检查,无明显异常发现。多次住院治疗,各专科给予相应治疗后症状无明显改善。遂来我科就诊,诊断为"焦虑障碍"。首次临床躯体症状分类量表评估提示抑制性躯体症状 1.08 分,激惹性躯体症状 1.71 分,生物性躯体症状 0.2 分,想象性躯体症状 1.8 分,认知性躯体症状 1.29 分,大五人格问卷测查提示神经质 3.9,外倾性 3.4,开放性 2.8,宜人性 3,严谨性 3.2。给予度洛西汀 60～120mg/d,喹硫平 100～200mg/d,氯硝西泮 0～3mg/d 治疗,辅以心理治疗。

治疗 4 周后患者开始感觉手脚麻木的症状明显好转,有肌肉跳动的感觉但不影响生活。评估临床躯体症状分类量表提示抑制性躯体症状 0.08 分,激惹性躯体症状 0.70 分,生物性躯体症状 0 分,想象性躯体症状 0.80 分,认知性躯体症状 0.21 分。治疗 3 个月后患者自述情绪稳定,麻木感完全消失,偶有肌肉跳动感,"自己完全是个正常人了"。评估临床躯体症状分类量表提示抑制性躯体症状 0 分,激惹性躯体症状 0.14 分,生物性躯体症状 0 分,想象性躯体症状 0.20 分,认知性躯体症状 0.14 分。

实验室检查: 首次内分泌检查结果提示:TSH 0.857mU/L,T_3 1.52nmol/L,T_4 101.5nmol/L,FT_3 4.32pmol/L,FT_4 18.63pmol/L,ACTH 44.64pmol/L,皮质醇 632.8nmol/L。经过 3 个月治疗后末次内分泌检查结果:TSH 2.44mU/L,T_3 1.89nmol/L,T_4 119.8nmol/L,FT_3 5.52pmol/L,FT_4 17.62pmol/L,ACTH 19.30pmol/L,皮质醇 503.6nmol/L。

治疗者体会: 从症状学角度分析,该患者的症状具有如下特点:①躯体症状具有多部位、多样性的特点。②各专科均未发现恰当的躯体疾病解释，于专科处理后症状也无改善。③症状影响患者的社会功能。④患者同时具有精神方面的症状，如睡眠差，心慌、坐立不安。对于具有类似特征的患者应考虑焦虑障碍的可能性。患者手脚发麻酸胀、肌肉跳动的感觉等方面的躯体症状理应考虑为"激惹性躯体症状"。

另外，患者在病程中也出现了焦虑的认知改变，最突出的问题是灾难性思维，觉得自己得了大病，四处求医，并且天气变化时症状加重，且症状越来越多样化。经临床躯体症状分类量表筛查后提示为想象性和激惹性躯体症状，给予推荐方案中的抗焦虑药+非典型抗精神病药物，辅以心理治疗，疗效明显，3个月后复评临床躯体症状分类量表想象性和激惹性躯体症状评分显著下降，患者感觉良好。因此，我们在遇到有躯体症状的患者时，应全面分析、评估症状，以便合理选用治疗方案。此外，对于躯体症状分类量表结果的解读，除了关注排列在第一的主要症状外，还应该关注提示其余几个症状成分的得分情况，特别应该注意得分第二位的症状成分。该案例中激惹性躯体症状得分第一，而认知性躯体症状得分第二，故 SNRI 类药物+非典型抗精神病药物为主的治疗方案应该是取得疗效的关键。

五、以疼痛为主要特征的激惹性躯体症状案例

患者杨某，女性，55 岁，因"全身疼痛 3 年，加重伴蚁爬感 2 个月"入风湿免疫科。患者 3 年前出现四肢肌肉疼痛，行走受限，伴手足麻木，在笔者所在医院查抗核抗体 ++1：1000，补体 C3 0.6970 g/L；骨密度检查示骨质疏松；唇腺活检示下唇黏膜轻度慢性炎，伴鳞状上皮增生，仅见一分叶状小唾液腺组织，部分唾液腺腺泡减少，消失伴纤维组织增生，在笔者所在医院诊断为"干燥综合征、骨质疏松"，给予泼尼松、茴三硫片等治疗后，以上症状明显缓解。1 年前，患者无明显诱因出现右侧胸背痛，与呼吸无关，且长期失眠，笔者所在医院诊断为"干燥综合征；纤维肌痛综合征；脑白质脱髓鞘；肺部感染；骨质疏松"，予以泼尼松、甲泼尼龙、环磷酰胺、普瑞巴林、头孢美唑，以及补钙、护胃、改善微循环等对症支持治疗后好转出院。2 个

月前患者再次出现全身肌肉及关节疼痛并伴蚁爬感，行走受限，伴手足麻木，头痛头晕，失眠严重。入风湿免疫科后按干燥综合征治疗无明显疗效。转入笔者所在科行临床躯体症状分类量表评估，结果为：激惹性躯体症状因子分 2.93，抑制性躯体症状因子分 2.92，想象性躯体症状因子分 2.40，生物性躯体症状因子分 1.60，认知性躯体症状因子分 1.30。查甲状腺功能、皮质醇、促肾上腺皮质激素、性激素、糖耐量试验均在正常范围。按激惹性躯体症状分类给予度洛西汀、硫必利、奥氮平、氯硝西泮等治疗。治疗 1 个月后症状明显减轻，激惹性躯体症状因子分 1.85，抑制性躯体症状因子分 2.00，想象性躯体症状因子分 1.60，生物性躯体症状因子分 0.80，认知性躯体症状因子分 0.93。治疗 2 个月后诉疼痛几乎消失，仅兴趣还未完全恢复。目前尚在继续治疗中。

治疗体会：此患者虽确诊为干燥综合征，但全身疼痛症状不能以干燥综合征解释，不应局限于生物学治疗。按心身医学理论，患者的全身疼痛症状、蚁爬感属于激惹性躯体症状，按临床躯体症状分类量表评估结果为：激惹性躯体症状因子分和抑制性躯体症状因子分居于前两位，故应按情绪性躯体症状治疗，给予度洛西汀、硫必利、奥氮平、氯硝西泮的联合治疗方案，患者疗效良好。

六、以类幻觉症状为特征的想象性躯体症状案例

患者黄某，男性，55 岁，舞蹈演员。4 年前开始出现感全身关节松散、移位，当运动时感觉脊柱被拉伸长了，肩胛骨部位有关节位置改变，局部肌肉被牵拉、酸软不适，并感觉血液在血管里滚动，因此不敢活动。当时到神经外科就诊，做腰部 X 线片及颈肩 MRI 检查未见异常。患者开始整日为上述躯体不适而忧虑，并伴有阵发性手心发热、出汗、心慌。3 年多前至华西医院心理卫生中心，诊断"精神分裂症"，服用利培酮 5mg/d，奥氮平每晚 2.5mg，感躯体不适缓解不理想，因活动后感觉躯体不适更明显而终日躺在床上，并渐渐感觉从脚部往上至头顶的肌肉在游走性旋转，骨骼肌肉松散。遂到笔者所在医

院住院，诊断"躯体形式障碍"，首次临床躯体症状分类量表提示抑制性躯体症状 0.75 分，激惹性躯体症状 1.21 分，生物性躯体症状 0.20 分，想象性躯体症状 2.60 分，认知性躯体症状 1.00 分；大五人格问卷测试提示神经质 1.83，外倾性 4.25，开放性 3.17，宜人性 3.67，严谨性 4.17。给予度洛西汀 60～120mg/d，喹硫平 200～800mg/d，坦度螺酮 15～30mg/d 治疗，辅以心理治疗及暗示治疗，治疗 4 周后患者开始感觉"有微妙变化"，担忧减轻，肌肉旋转感逐渐不影响活动，评估临床躯体症状分类量表提示抑制性躯体症状 0 分，激惹性躯体症状 0.07 分，生物性躯体症状 0 分，想象性躯体症状 1.67 分，认知性躯体症状 0.29 分。治疗 3 个月后患者自述情绪稳定，躯体不适明显减轻，偶尔感背部肌肉在扭转，但活动如常，评估临床躯体症状分类量表提示抑制性躯体症状 0 分，激惹性躯体症状 0.07 分，生物性躯体症状 0 分，想象性躯体症状 1.30 分，认知性躯体症状 0.14 分。

实验室检查：首次内分泌检查结果提示：TSH 3.997mU/L，T_3 1.207nmol/L，T_4 90.606nmol/L，FT_3 5.241pmol/L，FT_4 14.218pmol/L，ACTH 40.28pmol/L，皮质醇 566.2nmol/L。经过 3 个月治疗后末次内分泌检查结果：TSH 4.259mU/L，T_3 0.987nmol/L，T_4 54.068nmol/L，FT_3 5.344pmol/L，FT_4 8.509pmol/L，ACTH 19.20pmol/L，皮质醇 439.2nmol/L。

治疗者体会：该患者躯体症状表现为肌肉骨骼松散、扭转，首次诊断为"精神分裂症"，是将此症状解读为内脏性幻觉，但经单纯抗精神病药物治疗效果欠理想，分析其症状，性质多变，且部位多处转移、不固定，结合其人格基础，患者系舞蹈演员，平素情感丰富、表演性强，经躯体症状量表筛查后提示为想象性躯体症状。想象性躯体症状主要源于暗示与自我暗示，其产生既与认知功能异常有关，也与负性情绪相关，因此给予抗焦虑药+非典型抗精神病药物治疗，辅以暗示治疗，疗效明显优于单纯使用抗精神病药物治疗。3 个月后复评临床躯体症状分类量表，想象性躯体症状评分下降。另外，患者在感到肌肉骨骼扭转时，并发了焦虑情绪，从首次评估中筛查出激惹性躯体症状可看出，这也是使用抗焦虑药物的依据，经治疗焦虑情绪缓解良好，3个月后复评，激惹性症状评分明显下降。故在解读躯体症状的时候，重要的是更为全面、综合地把握患者症状实质。同时，使用适当的工具，如躯体症状量表及人格测量可以帮助我们定性症状，也可量化评估疗效及预后。

七、具有节律特征的抑制性躯体症状案例

患者刘某，女性，27岁。因"反复意识丧失、四肢抽搐10年余，情绪低落，兴趣下降5年"前来就诊。患者10年余前被确诊为癫痫，发作形式以全面强直阵挛发作为主，频率2~3次/月。曾使用卡马西平、丙戊酸钠、左乙拉西坦等药物治，10余年来反复调整药物效果不佳。5年前患者逐渐出现情绪低落，对事物兴趣减退，并出现以早醒为主的睡眠障碍，白天精神较差，感全身乏力，经常出现自杀观念；且月经周期长期不规律，在外院诊断为多囊卵巢综合征（PCOS）。上述症状已经严重影响患者的社会功能，因此10年前便辞职在家治病。患者在神经内科住院期间内科查体及神经系统检查均未见异常；辅助检查：长程视频脑电图（VEEG）提示重度异常；甲状腺功能：TSH↑；汉密尔顿抑郁量表（HAMD）得分为22分。首次行临床躯体症状分类量表评估结果提示：抑制性躯体症状2.4分，激惹性躯体症状1.9分，生物性躯体症状1.6分，想象性躯体症0.9分，认知性躯体症状1.3分，提示该患者以抑制性躯体症状为主，在治疗上给予丙戊酸钠500mg bid、左乙拉西坦500mg bid、西酞普兰20mg qd等药物治疗。1个月后患者情绪明显好转，癫痫发作频率由上个月3次减为1次；在月经3~5天完善性激素、甲状腺功能、血脂全套、OGTT及妇科彩超检查均未见明显异常；复查HAMD得分由22分减为14分，躯体症状量表总分由8.1分减为2.3分。对其疗效的总体评估应视为"显效"。目前在继续维持治疗中。

治疗者体会： 对该患者使用的基本治疗方案为抗癫痫药物（心境稳定剂）+SSRI类药物，而治疗效果是抑郁情绪、癫痫发作和多囊卵巢综合征无论从生物学指标、抑郁体验还是作为负性感受的躯体症状

均得到明显改善。这不得不联想到三者之间理应存在某种内在联系的可能性。复习国外相关研究文献提示，病理性抑郁心境属于情感节律的异常，癫痫属于中枢神经系统电生理节律的异常，而多囊卵巢综合征则源于 HPA 轴节律的异常，作为主要心境稳定剂的抗癫痫类药物对稳定和调整生物节律具有重要作用，三类情况同时缓解的关键应该在于这种生物节律调整的核心作用，而 SSRI 类药物在此例患者的治疗中也起到了重要的辅助作用。由此案例应该联想到的问题是在临床诊疗中，应该关注节律障碍的问题，同时，对于躯体症状分类来说，应该在今后的临床实践中注意是否专门存在"节律性躯体症状"的可能性。

八、具有节律特征的激惹性躯体症状案例

患者肖某，男性，15 岁，初三在读。因"反复腹痛 5 个月"入院。5 个月前患者参加军训 1 天后出现呕吐胃内容物，每天 3～4 次，无其他伴随症状。于当地医院按"急性胃肠炎"对症处理，7 天后呕吐好转，开始出现腹痛，为中上腹及左侧腹部持续性绞痛，无放射痛，进食后加剧，无伴随症状。行腹部平片考虑"肠梗阻？"，对症治疗后呕吐消失，疼痛持续存在。于华西医院消化科住院治疗，腹部彩超、全腹增强 CT、小肠钡餐未见明显异常；胃镜：胃体中段大弯侧见一片状红斑，肠镜：末段回肠炎，直肠炎；回肠末段病检：黏膜中度慢性炎，淋巴滤泡形成。消化内科全科讨论后考虑"紫癜性肠病"，予以甲泼尼龙冲击治疗，腹痛缓解后出院。1 周后再次出现腹痛，为左侧及中上腹固定性持续性疼痛，阵发性加剧，伴全腹压痛。入住消化科后再次予以皮质激素治疗，症状未见明显缓解。转至笔者所在科。辅助检查：三大常规，血常规白细胞计数 $3.32×10^9$/L↓，其余正常。肝肾功、大小便常规、心电图正常。皮质醇（8～10 点）11.26nmol/L↓。ACTH、甲功、甲状腺抗体、甲状腺彩超均正常。评估躯体症状：抑制性躯体症状 0.33 分，激惹性躯体症状 0.93 分，生物性躯体症状 0 分，想象性躯体症状 0.36 分，认知性躯体症状 0.7 分，总分 29 分。

使用度洛西汀 30mg tid，硫必利 100mg tid，奥氮平 5mg qn，丙戊酸钠 500mg qd 治疗，1 周后自诉腹痛症状消失，焦虑情绪及睡眠症状均得到明显改善，1 个月后腹痛症状无反复，复评抑制性躯体症状 0.08 分，激惹性躯体症状 0.21 分，生物性躯体症状 0 分，想象性躯体症状 0.07 分，认知性躯体症状 0.3 分，总分为 8 分。3 个月后呕吐症状无反复，复评抑制性躯体症状 0 分，激惹性躯体症状 0.07 分，生物性躯体症状 0 分，想象性躯体症状 0 分，认知性躯体症状 0.1 分，总分 2 分。复查内分泌示：TSH 1.930mU/L，T_3 1.4nmol/L，T_4 99.47nmol/L，FT_3 3.60pmol/L，FT_4 20.20pmol/L，ACTH 76.14pmol/L，PTC 397.60nmol/L。

　　治疗者体会：总结该患者诊疗过程，成败关键在于对患者躯体症状的解读缺乏大医学的理念，因此前期诊疗的挫折关键是仅去反复查找患者可能存在的病理损害而忽略了对患者症状性质的解读。采用躯体症状分类量表的评估结果提示该患者症状的性质是激惹性躯体症状，但仅限于此还是不够的，再次梳理病史资料发现了患者激惹性躯体症状具有节律性的特征，由此制订的治疗方案为心境稳定剂+SNRI类药物+非典型抗精神病药物，治疗目标为以心境稳定剂调整节律，以 SNRI 类药物抗焦虑和抑郁，以非典型抗精神病药物改善认知功能，故而取得良好效果。与案例七同理，该案例的诊疗过程提示是否存在单独的节律性躯体症状的可能，值得在今后的临床实践中进一步积累治疗案例。

九、想象性躯体症状伴随激惹性躯体症状案例

　　患者杨某，女性，56 岁，离退休人员。2 年前患者无明显诱因下出现入睡困难，因程度较轻，未予重视。其后逐渐感腹胀、腹痛，疼痛部位不固定，可放射至背部，腹痛严重时伴胃部发热、反酸，感头昏、心慌、多汗、四肢发麻，自述闭上眼时可减轻。小便正常，大便干结、便秘，长期服用"泻药"。多次于当地医院就诊，均未查及明确病理改变，患者自感症状严重，无法正常生活，四处求医。4 个月前外院考虑"肠粘连"，行"肠粘连松解术"后患者躯体不适无减轻。

3 个月前外院肠镜示：横结肠肝曲息肉样黏膜隆起（性质？），行"横结肠肝曲结肠息肉切除术"后症状仍无明显减轻。近两个月患者感腹痛等上述症状加重，伴排便困难、尿痛、尿不尽，进食后即有便意，但大便干结，难以解出。患者整日因躯体不适而担忧，入睡困难。入院查肝肾功能、血常规、大便常规、肿瘤标志物、腹部彩超均未见异常，皮质醇（8～10 点）663.6nmol/L。CT 全腹平扫：左侧输尿管轻度扩张，左侧肾盂密度稍高，尿盐结晶（请结合临床）？腹主动脉周围淋巴结稍增多。评估躯体症状：抑制性躯体症状 0.71 分，激惹性躯体症状 2 分，生物性躯体症状 0 分，想象性躯体症状 2.2 分，认知性躯体症状 0.71 分，总分为 66 分。予以度洛西汀 60mg bid，氯硝西泮 1mg tid 及莫沙必利 5mg tid 等药物治疗，辅以暗示治疗。1 个月后患者腹胀、腹痛、便秘、排尿困难症状明显好转，复评躯体症状：抑制性躯体症状 0.29 分，激惹性躯体症状 1 分，生物性躯体症状 0 分，想象性躯体症状 1.4 分，认知性躯体症状 0.43 分，总分为 36 分。

治疗者体会： 患者主要症状为疼痛，躯体症状量表评估结果显示想象性躯体症状评分最高，而想象性躯体症状产生的病理心理基础是暗示，暗示与认知功能密切相连，此外该患者的次高得分为激惹性躯体症状。正如在第一章和本章第二节所提到的那样，想象性躯体症状的治疗较之其他类型的躯体症状的治疗更趋个别化和多元化，而该患者的躯体症状量表次高得分为激惹症状，因此在综合治疗的基础上，将治疗目标集中于抗焦虑及对症治疗取得成功。通过该案例的治疗还应注意的是对躯体症状量表评估结果应该全面分析，而并非简单地仅看最高分。

十、以述情障碍为病理心理基础的激惹性躯体症状

患者曾某，女性，15 岁，学生。因"反复呕吐 7 年余，复发 2 天"入院。患者自诉 7 年多前无明显诱因出现呕吐，呕吐物为少量无酸味的胃内容物，发作前伴有明显中上腹部疼痛，伴有轻度恶心，不伴有发热、头痛、眩晕等；发作后感到疲乏，烦躁，进食后会加重呕

吐症状。呕吐一天以内发作数次，多在白天发作，呕吐最开始为少量胃内容物，后为呕吐清水样物质或干呕。遂到当地医院消化内科住院治疗，住院期间患者基本无法自己进食，进食后立即发生呕吐，只能靠输液维持基本营养，伴有睡眠差，主要为眠浅，易醒，给予一般对症支持治疗，一周后上述症状缓解。5 月余后患者无明显诱因再次出现上述症状，于四川大学华西附属第二医院住院治疗，辅助检查全身CT、MRI、胃镜、钡餐、三大常规等提示无明显异常，一周后自行缓解。5 月余前月经初潮后停止发作 2 年余。3 年多前再次出现发作性呕吐，平均 1～5 个月发作 1 次，多次外院诊断"自主神经功能紊乱性胃肠病"，每次均住院给予一般输液对症支持治疗，一般一周左右自行缓解，发作渐渐频繁，患者学习成绩虽然一直保持中等，但逐渐下降。患者为此感到焦虑。2 天多前患者再发上述症状，门诊以"神经性呕吐"收入笔者所在科。

　　入笔者所在科后诊断"焦虑障碍"，评估临床躯体症状分类量表示：抑制性躯体症状 0.33 分，激惹性躯体症状 0.93 分，生物性躯体症状 0 分，想象性躯体症状 0.7 分，认知性躯体症状 0.36 分。予艾司西酞普兰 10～20mg/d，奥氮平 25mg qn，丙戊酸钠 500mg qd，氯硝西泮 1mg bid 2mg qn。

　　治疗 1 周后患者自诉发作性呕吐症状消失，焦虑情绪及睡眠症状均得到明显改善。治疗 1 个月后呕吐症状无反复，复评临床躯体症状分类量表示：抑制性躯体症状 0.08 分，激惹性躯体症状 0.21 分，生物性躯体症状 0 分，想象性躯体症状 0.3 分，认知性躯体症状 0.07 分。治疗 3 个月后呕吐症状无反复，复评临床躯体症状分类量表示：抑制性躯体症状 0 分，激惹性躯体症状 0.07 分，生物性躯体症状 0 分，想象性躯体症状 0.1 分，认知性躯体症状 0 分。

　　实验室检查：入院查内分泌示：TSH 1.930mU/L，FT_3 3.60pmol/L，FT_4 20.20pml/L，T_3 0.99nmol/L，T_4 99.47nmol/L，ACTH 76.14ng/L，PTC 397.60nmol/L。经过 3 个月治疗后复查内分泌示：TSH 1.930mU/L，FT_3 3.60pmol/L，FT_4 20.20pmol/L，T_3 1.4nmol/L，T_4 99.47nmol/L，ACTH

76.14ng/L，PTC 397.60nmol/L。

　　治疗者体会：该患者的焦虑可解读为三个层面，躯体层面——器官功能紊乱的症状：腹痛、呕吐；体验层面——运动不安、交感神经兴奋的症状：心慌、坐立不安；认知层面——固执、刻板的行为或思考方式，不愿改变，焦虑情绪。评临床躯体症状分类量表患者显示为激惹性躯体症状，根据共识推荐，采用抗焦虑方案为主；结合患者情绪、行为、睡眠及内分泌等多种生物节律紊乱，加用丙戊酸钠稳定生物节律。在心理方面解读，该患者的症状具有以下成分。①述情障碍：患者在情绪的识别、情绪的表达方面的缺失导致她只能以躯体症状来表达自己不开心的情绪。②获益：原发性获益包括患者出现症状可逃避繁重的学业，在生病以后母亲对她的包容和要求降低为继发性获益。③广泛的性压抑：患者从小在标准化教育下长大，有着刻板的思维、生活方式，呕吐从这一角度可理解为广泛意义的性压抑。

（郭　菁　廖宗炳　陈佳佳　刘璨璨　阿茹晗　周亚玲　曾凡敏

孙学礼　耿　婷　著）

第五章　"共识"结论

就上述设想及所进行的一系列验证及研究工作而言，合作团队所进行的工作归纳起来包括：

（1）首次全面地、从心身医学的视角提出了临床躯体症状的 4 种分类，通过躯体症状分类工具的研制，为提出的分类理论假设提供了较为有力的支持性证据。

（2）通过实证研究，也就是直接寻证研究，对在心身医学理论框架基础上所研发的《西部精神医学协会（WCPA）临床躯体症状分类量表（第二版）》进行了信度、效度检验，结果显示自编分类工具具有较好的效标效度，可以试用于实际临床工作。

（3）对心身医学理论框架下的所研发的《西部精神医学协会（WCPA）临床躯体症状分类量表（第二版）》进行了多中心研究，对不同躯体症状的治疗疗效显著再次证明了本研究的理论构建的科学性和合理性，现场测量数据也再次吻合临床躯体症状分类量表的内部结构模型。临床测试的结果再次为本研究假设提供了证据，从而证实假设中四类临床躯体症状分类的存在，因此可试用于临床对躯体症状的识别中。

（4）多中心的研究证明了所推荐的对各类躯体症状的治疗方案行之有效，可作为医疗实践中的重要参考。

（5）通过心身医学理论下对临床躯体症状的解读，对慢性非感染性疾病治疗至少包括三个维度：一是病因学治疗维度，二是病理生理、病理心理治疗维度，三是症状学治疗维度。提示对躯体症状应予以更多关注。

（6）由于在临床对多中心研究中随访时间相对短，仅仅 3 个月结束随访。但 3 个月随访充分证明了治疗效果的显著，也为本项目症状分型的理论假设提供了依据。我们也将继续随访工作并将对随访结果进行报道，以进一步在更多的实践活动中验证我们的理论假设。此外，在自编问卷的工作中，本研究受试者数量相对不够大，大部分来自同一单位。因此可能存在选择性偏倚。我们也将继续修正和校正量表，降低选择性偏倚对研究结果的干扰。

（7）此为在 2014～2016 年的研究及实践中得出的共识，理念的形成及学术观点的发展是动态的和不断证伪的过程，在不断征求不同意见、不断扩大实践范围的过程中，还将得出今后数年不断完善的"共识"。

总之，对躯体症状的独立治疗应得到更多的关注。心身统一的观点及多元化的临床思维模式是认识躯体症状和治疗躯体症状的重要前提。

（孙学礼　曾凡敏　著）

Chapter 1 Related issues of somatic symptom classification under the theoretical framework of psychosomatic medicine

Section 1 Hypothesis of somatic symptom classification under psychosomatic medical theory

Clinical disciplines have to deal with various somatic symptoms of patients during consultation. Conventionally, the symptoms always come with corresponding pathological basis. Thus, the somatic symptoms provide a clue to various pathological changes and can serve as a starting point, or a fundamental basis for diagnosis and treatment. These symptoms are classified according to organ systems, such as symptoms of the digestive tract, respiratory symptom, cardiovascular symptom, and nervous system symptom. This approach helps a clinician decipher the clues and then manage the case through triage, examination, and come up with a treatment plan. There are several problems with this traditional way of thinking: first, the symptoms corresponding to a system of organs do not necessarily indicate that the particular system has problems. Therefore, when analysis of the symptoms points to a system and if no abnormalities are found, the diagnosis and treatment shall be halted. If the patient is referred to other department, this means a new diagnosis and treatment will be started, and it is a waste of time and resource. Second, some symptoms overlap in the classification of diseases; thus, it is difficult to pinpoint the affected organs. For example, vomiting can be classified as a digestive system symptom or also as a nervous system symptom. Third, a cause will lead to an effect, a mode of universal thinking can dominate clinical thinking. The fact is that a single cause may not necessarily lead to a specific consequence, while a consequence can be a result of many causes. The lack of diversity in thinking and the failure to consider a problem from multiple perspectives will lead to blindsided thinking in clinical and research work, having a negative effect on understanding the disease and formulating treatment plan. For example, if a patient had abdominal pain, menstrual disorders, and the examination found uterine myoma, so myomectomy surgery was given immediately. However, the patient still had pain after the operation, or even can't get out of bed, there was almost a medical dispute. But after the anti-anxiety treatment for 2-4 weeks, the pain disappeared, and patient discharged and came back to work. The case shows that although the symptoms appear in the lower abdomen, but the problem lies in somewhere else (psychological other than physical), which at least indicated that there are many causes could lead to the patient's pain, but only treatment for one system definitely can't reach the expected results.

Clinical classification and diagnosis are intended to target treatment, and also to generate correct ideas for clinical diagnosis and treatment. As mentioned above, adherence to the conventional system that is designed to decipher somatic symptoms in the traditional way can lead to drawbacks and misconceptions. The International Association for the Study of Pain in 1979 defined pain as "an unpleasant sensory and emotional experience associated with actual or potential tissue damage or described in terms of such damage". This definition stresses the importance of the emotional and suffering aspects of clinical somatic symptoms. As recognized and understood according to the above definition, a physical symptom is essentially a "feeling" , and this kind of "feeling" is related to "damage" or "potential damage", and it is associated with the subjective experience of the individual. In other words, a physical symptom may not have a purely biological source, but it is always related to cognition, emotion, personality, and other psychological elements. Based on this idea, somatic symptoms can also be defined as follows:

A. Somatic symptoms are organic reactions to the emotion

This definition comes from the theory of alexithymia and "secondary gain". The definition "unconsciousness" mentioned above is needed to elaborate these 2. Organ function change in the expression of the demands exists in biosphere is an universal phenomenon, such as small animals have urinary incontinence out of fear or muscle tremors; when you say "I'm sick of you" . is also the changes of organ function "expression of demand". Because the evolution and development of the human nervous system, expression of demand in the human is mainly verbal or emotional, if in some individuals will change organ function as an expression of "the main way to demand", this is called "alexithymia". An 18 year old woman with severe vomiting was admitted 7 times within 1 year, the symptom relieved very quickly during each admission, but repeated attacks occurred. The examination found no pathological causes of vomiting. After inquiring the medical history and the current state of mind, we found that the patient had a crush on her elder brother, and this might be the cause for vomiting (emotional aversion). Psychological counseling and anti-anxiety treatment were given and the symptom disappeared, and the 2 years follow up found no occurrence. The case is the best example of physical symptoms that appear as the expression of demand. If unconsciously using their own physical dysfunction as the "chips" of actual benefits, this is a condition known as "secondary benefit". As the conversion of the pathological basis based on psychological barriers is the best example.

B. The somatic symptom is an important way to relieve the inner conflict

The symptom is a bridge connecting the body and mind, the individual is often not aware of their own deep inner conflict, which induces somatic symptoms. In the battle with external environment, the body finally collapses and signals the need of the intervention. This course is latent and at the subconscious level, but later there might be physical symptoms and thus such inner conflict will surface, which is not a threat to the individual's self-image but protection over the individual spirit from collapse, and also "protest" real life pressure. In this conflict, the patients could not express his direct conflict, only through somatic symptoms, symbolically the conflict to swallow. A fox came to the grape vine and wanted to eat some grapes, but it couldn't climb. The fox had options: one is to climb, which means to force yourself to do things that you can't achieve, the other one is to quit, which means if you are reluctant, you have to admit that there is always something out of your reach. However, the fox took a third option that worked: "the grapes are too sour to eat". This is the best explanation of mental defense mechanism of rationalization. Similarly, this applies to when a student wants to get an A but he is not an A student. There are two options: one is to achieve the first place by working hard; the other one is give up, which means he must admit that he is a A student. The way to solve this problem is "because I was sick, so I can't become an A student". The somatic symptoms became a way to ease the conflict.

C. Somatic symptom is the emotion itself

Somatic symptoms are unpleasant subjective experience. If somatic symptoms are defined as emotion itself, which are mainly negative. Clinically, the negative emotion is referring to anxiety and depression. In the case of anxiety, clinical interpretation of anxiety is the inner experience of disturbance or fear associated with autonomic nervous system function disorder and motor restlessness, so anxiety is involved in the physical state, the experience and cognition. Anxiety is a basic human emotion, which maintains the necessary vigilance, this is directly related to self-defense. Typical symptom that increased awareness and self-defense is a pain. In addition, organ function disturbance or symptom such as urinary frequency, urgency and irritable bowel syndrome are technically fall into this category.

D. The somatic symptoms is negative interpretation of the individual to the body feeling

This definition means that cognitive system plays a major role in those with somatic symptoms. Various feelings exist at any time, through cognitive effects, if the individual has a feeling as a positive interpretation has and this becomes the individual's current feeling, if negative interpretation, this feeling is not what an individual wants, then come somatic symptoms. Take the pain as an example, when the time of negative interpretation, the pain has become one of the most common clinical symptoms, but people sometimes also in pursuit of the feeling of pain, or even think that it is "cool", for example, in the health care massage. At this time the pain is a symptom disturbs an individual, but a kind of enjoyable feeling.

E. The somatic symptoms are the result of learning or imitation

This definition mainly shows under the circumstances of suggestion or autosuggestion, individuals can reproduce the symptoms or copying the previous symptoms.

The implication is that the individual under the certain environment and the emotional atmosphere of influence from the outside of the unconditional acceptance, and in certain environments and certain emotional atmosphere of influence from their unconditional acceptance is called self suggestion. Suggestion and autosuggestion are the characteristics of human psychology, previous studies showed that they reach to the highest point at 5-7 years ago, and are higher in female than male; they might reduce age: But with the growth of age, the individual is suggestive remains and doesn't match with age, it is high-risk mental factor of somatic symptoms. In this case, the suggestion or implication is not about pathological damage but abnormal indication. In addition, the definition suggests, minors, the elderly, young people have the same symptoms of psychological meaning is different.

If the above definition is established, we can say the physical symptoms are not only indicating the physical illness but the evidence for mental diseases, mental disorders and personality traits.

Section 2   Specific recommendations for psychosomatic classification of somatic symptoms

According to the above explanation of somatic symptoms, there shall be two components of somatic symptoms in patients, even in the patients with body disease, one is "biological component", such as symptoms induced by tumor pathological changes, while the other at this time being called "a psychological component". Using the theory of psychosomatic medicine to interpret the clinical somatic symptoms shows that there is a guiding role of diversified mode of thinking in clinical work. Inertia thinking on medicine is unitary mode of thinking, in other words, somatic symptoms. Clinicians always intend to find the reason only from the angle of pathological damage and give the corresponding treatment, while ignoring the "psychological component", so the somatic symptoms have not been resolved satisfactorily, and it is worth noting that somatic symptoms are important to the mentality of the patients, quality of life, treatment compliance and prognosis. In addition, the law of sufficient reason suggests that there should be inevitable logical link between premises and conclusion. If there are symptoms, and at the same time the damage also exists, but judgment about causal relationship of symptoms and the damage is lacking of sufficient reason. It shall be noted and corrected if there is inertia thinking of clinical medicine. Interpretation of somatic symptoms with psychosomatic medicine provided a clinical basis for a comprehensive analysis of somatic symptoms and the different individuals of the same symptoms. Then, according to the psychosomatic medicine of somatic symptoms of interpretation, there are at least three dimensions in the treatment of chronic non infectious diseases, the first is the etiological treatment, the second is the pathophysiology, psychopathology, and the third is the symptom treatment. Therefore, the independent treatment of somatic symptoms needs more attention.

As the need for separate treatment of somatic symptoms, according to the above interpretation and comprehensive evaluation from psychosomatic medicine, physical symptoms can be basically classified as follows:

Biological somatic symptoms

These symptoms mainly are the nerve-ending stimulation induced by the local tissue lesion caused by physical, chemical, and biological factors or biochemical reactions caused by the suboptimal stimulation of nerve endings. This symptom is not based on the types and intensity of the stimulus, but the ascending pathway of nervous system is activated and descending pathway is inhibited. It is worth noting that the activation and transfer pathway inhibition blocked off not only from the biological pathway damage, can also be due to the changes, even derived from the state of mind, such as fight or other state of passion, there might be un-noted pain. This shows that whether biological damage can produce nega-tive feelings or what feeling is closely related to psychological factors.

Emotional somatic symptoms

In this case, the somatic experience is rooted in negative emotional symptoms. According to the theory of alexithymia, somatic symptoms are organic reactions to the emotion. In general, the reaction is from a nega-tive emotion, especially depression and anxiety. The "emotional" symp-toms can be divided into "inhibitive emotional symptoms" and "irritable mood symptoms". As the name suggests, the former mainly refers to the organ function is inhibited, such as anorexia, satiety, dizziness, uncon-sciousness. The most topical inhibition of somatic symptoms is functional dyspepsia; the latter is dysfunction, such as pain irritable bowel syndrome and other symptoms induced by irritation.

Cognitive somatic symptoms

The word "cognition" here has two meanings; one refers to the interpreta-tion of body awareness. Many types of somatic feelings are always pre-sent, but it is only when an individual has a negative interpretation of some feeling at the cognitive level that this feeling may become a somatic symptom. When people are having health care massage when feeling tired, many of them would ask a little strength, and get comfortable and relaxed feeling, in this case, the pain is needed at the cognitive level, the pain is known as "positive" interpretation, and when the pain is negative and the information at that time is a sort of "warning signal" for injury, i.e. somatic symptoms. An illusion in psychiatry is defined as a situation in which there is no objective stimulus, but stimulation of the sensory nerves in an organ is present, causing the perceptual experience corresponding to the organ. The second meaning of cognitive somatic symptoms is that some physical symptoms match the definition of an illusion. For example, bilateral tinnitus can be diagnosed and treated as an illusion. The characteristics of cognitive somatic symptoms are relatively fixed in their characteristics and location, and the symptoms are clear. As a middle-aged female patient admitted due to limp, the reason is because when walking the right foot feels like stepping on a pointy pebble of pigeon egg size and the pain induces the limp. The symptom disappeared after atypical antipsychotic treatment for two weeks.

Imaginative somatic symptoms

This category refers to the symptoms that resulted from imagination, suggestion, or autosuggestion. The typical characteristics of these symptoms are various and surreal. A young female patient had this feeling that she had multiple episodes of their "brain" was peeled off layer by layer. She was horrified and went to the doctor's complaining that she had the feeling that the brain cell peeled off to the knee joints or ankles where was an attack.

The significance of classification of somatic symptoms lies in: ①to develop clinical thinking and improve understanding of physical symptoms to better implement the unified psychosomatic point of view; ②to help establish guidelines for the diagnosis of somatic symptoms and mental illness; ③to help establish guidelines for the treatment of somatic symptoms, such as management of weakness with antidepressant treatments, irritable emotional symptoms with anti-anxiety drugs. Cognitive symptoms can be alleviated with cognitive-behavioral therapy, and biological symptoms by means of local and systemic physical treatment. It is worth noting that the methods intended to increase understanding of physical symptoms from more perspectives should vary from patient to patient and implement a thinking mode of diversification. Nevertheless, the unified psychosomatic point of view and diverse clinical thinking modes are aimed at identifying somatic symptoms and important prerequisites for the treatment of these symptoms. The pain could be an irritable physical symptom or just imaginary. In clinical practice, the current diseases, medical history, life experience, personality and emotional factors shall be taken into consideration. Even for the local damage or potential damage caused by the treatment of biological physical symptoms for which attention shall be paid to the non-biological factors. Even in the presence of the biological changes, determinants of physical symptoms are not only biological ones. As a kind of injury, the pain in some patients may last only a few days, and a few years for others. In a word, the psychosomatic unity and clinical thinking mode of diversification is an important prerequisite for understanding physical symptoms and treatment of somatic symptoms.

(Xueli Sun)

Chapter 2　Development of WCPA Somatic Symptom Classification Scale (WCPA-SSCS) under the theoretical framework of psycho-somatic medicine

Section 1　Revision of the theoretical dimensions of WCPA-SSCS

Clinical tests at the scene of the 2014-2015, we collected the using feedback of "classification scale of WCPA clinical somatic symptoms", mainly reflected in ①on emotional symptoms subdivision is not clear; ②reflects the rhythm of symptoms is not clear; ③about the symptoms described not enough language specification. Due to the sampling site and limitation of sampling time, in the process of field test in 2015-2016 we revised the emotional symptoms items, which embodied in the emotional somatic symptoms of irritable somatic symptoms and inhibitory somatic symptoms on the identification of not too clear, therefore, in the 2015 version, modify the item "4, 5, 29, 32, 39, 41", and emphasize the description of the inhibitory somatic symptoms. We adjusted the items in the first edition 4, 5, 29, 32, 41, specific content is as follows (Table 2-1-1):

Table 2-1-1   WCPA-SSCS with the original items control

The original item	The modified item
4. Body or limbs weakness or feel fatigue easily	4. Hysteresie symptoms(say less and less dynamic even stupor)
5. Choke with resentment	5. Can't give meaning to life
29. Easily tired after waking	29. Symptoms of morning heavy and sunset light
32. Feel their energy decline, slowing activity	32. Without a sense of worth
39. No interest to do something	39. No interest to do something (not with energy down)
41. Head heaviness or tightness	41. Limb lead feeling

First, process of amendment to scale

A. Objective

We carried out this scale revision work in Sichuan point. The group of patients using the adjusted scale test, included 478 cases (include exclusion standard in this project, see section 2 of this chapter), the male to female ration of 1: 1.4, the average age was 38.1±2.1 years old.

The inclusion criteria: ①male and female aged 18-65 years old; ②the regardless of existing diagnosis, non single somatic complaints in patients with various chronic non-infectious diseases in the patients with somatic symptoms; ③The patients concern about , or cause pain, or social function is affected, three in one.

The exclusion criteria: ①acute infection, acute trauma, perioperation period, chronic disease in acute stage patients; ②the critically ill or dying can not participate in the study; ③the pregnant or lactating women ④substance abuse.

B. The research content and methods

We use exploratory factor analysis and confirmation factor analysis method to inspect the internal structure of the changed classification scale, through the reliability and validity of the classification scale. Research tools including SPSS 19.0, adopted by the software of "SEM" R, "proc calis online" and LISTEL professional software SAS software.

C. The results of the study

a. The reliability assessment

We retested the scale after a week, the retest reliability as follows (Table 2-1-2):

Table 2-1-2   The retest reliability of revised items in WCPA-SSCS

Type of symptoms	α coefficient	Half coefficient
Emotional somatic symptoms	0.704	0.815
Inhibitory somatic symptoms	0.613	0.652
Irritable	0.543	0.622
Biological somatic symptoms	0.614	0.571
Imagine somatic symptoms	0.836	0.857
Cognitive somatic symptoms	0.691	0.650
Total	0.863	0.893

Results show that the overall five categories of testing reliability, measuring tool has good stability.

b. Validity evaluation

Tests at the scene of the 2015-2016, we have inspected the internal structure of adjusted scale. Entries after the classification of the scale adjustment for the exploratory factor analysis, gravel figure shows 55 items will be aggregated into five types are the most concentrated information. As shown in figure (Figure 2-1-1):

Results showed that 55 items will be aggregated into five types are the most scientific, the results and the scale revised prominent the difference between irritable somatic symptom and inhibitory somatic symptoms have consistency, to form a more clear concept of five classification of psychosomatic symptoms.

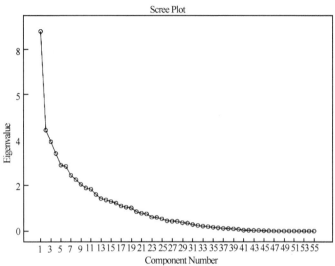

Figure 2-1-1   Scree plot

c. Confirmatory factor analysis

Tests at the scene of the 2015-2016 into the group of patients, we carried on the inspection of this classification scale. Through the confirmatory factor analysis of the adjustment items, which discuss data fitting degree, we get the following result (Figure 2-1-2):

Result suggests that path graph can be seen that the overall validity is good, all indicators meet the requirements of statistics. Especially the latent variables correlation coefficient between inhibitory somatic symptoms and irritable somatic symptoms is good.

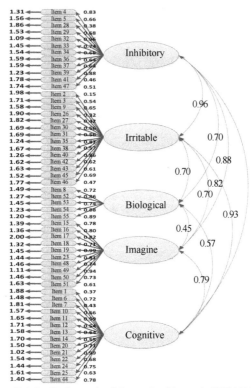

Figure 2-1-2   Path graph of the revised items in WCAP-SSCS

Second, the results of revised the scale

a. Based on the revised the clinical classification scale of WCPA somatic symptoms, the revised items for inhibitory somatic symptoms and irritable somatic symptoms have good identification.

b. Clinical test data in 2015-2016 to reflect the good internal structure of the adjusted scale, the fit of data is good.

c. We completed the WCPA clinical classification scale of somatic symptoms (revised). On whether the symptoms associated with the rhythm becomes an independent symptoms, as well as "scale" can reflect and related symptoms, such as problems for further exploration of the rhythms and revision.

Section 2   The instruction of WCPA-SSCS (second edition) under the theoretical framework of psychosomatic medicine

1. The scale introduction

a. According to the various aspects of the work which has been described previously, we finally research and develop WCPA somatic symptoms rating scale which is for clinical somatic symptoms classification, formed the WCPA-SSCS (second edition) and we declared national invention patent. (Patent Number: 201410363067.1).

b. WCPA-SSCS (second edition) includes 55 items in total, each entry has five scores. It contains two parts: one is self-evaluation by patient themselves (p) and the other is peer assessment by physicians (d).

c. Adaptation: this scale applies to chronic non-infectious diseases and evaluate the patients who are 18-65 years old, and patients with.

d. It is used to evaluate the severity of somatic symptoms in 4 weeks.

e. It excludes infectious disease and acute exacerbation of chronic disease.

2. Content of WCPA-SSCS (second edition)

A. Instruction

a. It lists some symptoms which is the symptoms the people may have, please read each one carefully, and then rate your degree those issues which have affected you or made you feel distressed in two weeks recently, fight "√" in the corresponding column.

b. Noting: the number 0 represents "not present", 1 means "mild", 2 means "moderate", 3 means "sever", 4 means "very serious", the larger the number, the higher the degree of rate.

B. Content

WCPA Somatic Symptoms Rating Scale (second edition)

Symptoms in recent four weeks	0 not present	1 mild	2 moderate	3 severe	4 very severe
1. Foreing body sensation in the throat or dysphagia; e					
2. Pain; b					
3. Sweat; b					
4. Body or limbs weakness or feel fatigue easily; a					
5. Choke with resentment; a					
6. Feel muscle movement; e					
7. Your symptoms are relatively fixed, clear, vivid; e					
8. .Patients with subjective discomfort experience; c					
9. Feel chills or hot in hands or foot; b					
10. Buzzing in brain or tinnitus; e					
11. Amnesia; e					
12. Can't concentrate; e					
13. Can't think fast or mind blank; e					
14. Hallucinations similar symptoms; e					
15. Thinking his or her body have serious problems; d					
16. Experiencing physical discomfort shift in various parts of the body; d					
17. Easy to experience the body disconfortable; d					
18. There are many different types of symptoms disturb you; d					
19. You can't accept that your doctor told you have no disease; d					
20. Precordial discomfort; e					

Continued

Symptoms in recent four weeks	0 not present	1 mild	2 moderate	3 severe	4 very severe
21. Transient unconsciousness; e					
22. Dizziness or vertigo; e					
23. Feel a part of the body loss function; d					
24. Feel hypoxia; e					
25. Systemic or localized swelling sense; e					
26. Difficulty falling asleep; b					
27. Shallow sleep; b					
28. Early awakening; a					
29. Easily tired after waking; a					
30. Dreaminess; b					
31. Frequent micturition; b					
32. without any power sense; a					
33. Loss of libido; a					
34. Indigestion; a					
35. Skin allergies; b					
36. Constipation; a					
37. Flatulence; a					
38. Ulcer; b					
39. No interest to do something; a					
40. Epigastric burning sensation; b					
41. Head heaviness or tightness ; a					
42. Diarrhea; b					
43. Nausea or vomiting; b					
44. Nasal foreign body sensation; e					
45. Palpitation; b					
46. Restlessness usually; b					
47. Feel something familiar becomes unfa- miliar or not really; a					
48. More sensitive to pain than others; d					

Consensus for Psychosomatic Classification, Diagnosis and Treatment
of Somatic Symptoms

Continued

Symptoms in recent four weeks	0 not present	1 mild	2 moderate	3 severe	4 very severe
49. Experiencing physical symptoms are diversity and variability; d					
50. You are more worried about health than most people; d					
51. If a disease brought to your attention, such as by radio, television, newspapers or someone you know, you worry about developing the disease, or link their discomfort associated with it ; d					
52. Medical laboratory examination; c					
53. Diseases with definite diagnosis; c					
54. Positive signs from doctors' examinations; c					
55. Visible damage; c					

3. The introduction of rating scale assessment

A. Example of using the scale

According to the medical record and site visits, please complete the scale score of 55 items. You can directly after each item corresponds to the symptom scores column tick.

For example: in the medical record, "item 1. the throat foreign body sensation or difficulty swallowing". Classification according to your estimate, or see the somatic symptoms scale using manual.

(Excerpts) scale using manual:

Item 1. the throat foreign body sensation or difficulty swallowing:

Level 0: without the symptoms;

Level 1: 2 weeks in 1 to 2 times, almost don't cause pain feeling;

Level 2: 1 to 2 times appear in one week, a little pain;

Level 3: symptoms appear every day in a week, pain is obvious;

Level 4: very obvious symptoms appeared several times a day, very obvious pain.

Comprehensive evaluation: what do you think of the case the symptoms as "mild", corresponding in item 1 "mild" column "tick", as shown in the figure below:

Symptoms in recent four weeks	0 not present	1 mild	2 moderate	3 severe	4 very severe
1. Foreing body sensation in the throat or Dysphagia; e		√			
2. Pain; b					
3. Sweat; b					

And so on, complete the score of 55 items.

After you complete 55 project detailed score, please according to the questionnaire results calculation method(see attachment), can get the physical symptom main types of the medical record and the secondary type, the result can be one of them as reference in clinical diagnosis and treatment of somatic symptoms.

B. Rating scale details

This rating scale assessment by self-evaluation or peerassessment. Item 52, 53, 54, 55 are evaluated by doctors, and the others are self-evaluation. The details are following:

a. The self-evaluation 5 degree introduction:

Item 1, 2, 3, 4, 5, 6, 9, 10, 11, 12, 13, 14, 20, 21, 22, 23, 24, 25, 34, 35, 36, 37, 40, 41, 42, 43, 44, 45, 46, 47 items:

Score 0: no symptoms;

Score 1: once or twice within two weeks, almost do not cause pain sensation;

Score 2: once or twice within one week, with a slight pain;

Score 3: obviously feel pain once a day within a week;

Score 4: feel seriously painful several times every day.

b. Item 7: your symptoms are relatively fixed, clear, vivid; here speak of "symptoms" is defined as any physical symptoms, such as itching, swelling and pain, based on this, the following rating:

Score 0: no fixed, clear symptoms;

Score 1: physical symptoms are relative fix, clear, with a slight pain;

Score 2: physical symptoms are fixed, clear with obvious pain;

Score 3: physical symptoms are fixed, clear with serious pain;

Score 4: physical symptoms are fixed, clear with very serious pain.

c. Item 8: patients' subjective uncomfortable experiences, connotation refers to subjective discomfort experienced no clear position, and without a clear systemic discomfort. Gets the first of the symptoms is based on a patient's thematic and, secondly, rater be judged according to describes the condition of the patient. After the symptom decision clear, based on the following items to score matter, specific scoring criteria for the items:

Score 0: patients have no obvious uncomfortable experience;

Score 1: patients experience a slight discomfort in a quiet environment, but are not aware of it when take an activity or work;

Score 2: the experience of patient with obvious discomfort, which does not affect the normal life and work;

Score 3: patients experience obvious discomfort, which affects the normal work and life;

Score 4: doctors observe significant painful experience, as a reference and evidence for the diagnosis of disease.

d. Item 15: thinking his or her body have serious problems; objective score according to the article information in two ways: one is the patient's own direct expression, second, clinicians according to in health care seeking behavior of patients with specific performance. For example, constantly asked to do body checks, but do not believe the neg-

ative of check results, or doubt the result of body checking is not serious than their actual situation. So, repeatedly seek diagnosis and
treatment, but raised questions about raised questions about the medical measures or do not agree with, or constantly pestered; patients
"disease concept", that is, apart from the disease, and can't think of
other problems, and nor do other daily activities. Objective score re-
quired on this article in the comprehensive availability of patient information to accurately judge. Specific rating looks this:

Score 0: do not consider any serious problems in physical;

Score 1: Although he knows his body has no big problem, but still have
concern because of physical discomfort;

Score 2: firmly believe that there are some problems in physical;

Score 3: believe that there are nearly serious problems in physical, and
want to make it better by medical treatment can;

Score 4: believe that there are extremely serious problems in physical,
and medical treatment may not able to make it better.

e. Item 16: experiencing physical discomfort shift in various parts of the
   body; set this item aims to understand whether there is no fixed does
   not apply to experience, "not" can include any negative experience,
   such as chills, fever, numbness and pain. Specific rating are follows:

Score 0: no migratory physical discomfort;

Score 1: physical discomfort is not fixed, and it appears about once or
twice every two weeks with a sense of a little pain;

Score 2: physical discomfort is not fixed, and it appears about once or
twice every week with a sense of moderate pain;

Score 3: physical discomfort migrates in different parts of body, and it
appears once a day with serious pain;

Score 4: physical discomfort migrates in different parts of body, and it
appears many times in a day with very serious pain.

f. Item 17: easy to experience the body disconfortable; item has two aspects meaning, one is refers to patients is easy experience to body discomfort able, or will this does not apply zoom. If he or she just woke up after sleeping a lot people can experience the feeling of heaviness, as patients complained of; the second is easy to body feeling made negative interpretation of this is normal, such as stools in front of minor abdominal pain, casual feel of the carotid arteries, specific grade, see the following criteria:

Score 0: not sensitive of the changing in various parts of the body, neither concern about it;

Score 1: concerned about the changes of the body, but no pain sensation;

Score 2: more concerned about the changes to the body and with some painful feelings;

Score 3: very concerned about the changes of the body with some obvious painful feeling; but attention is able to be shifted;

Score 4: extremely concerned about the changes of the body with heavy painful feeling; and attention is not able to be shifted.

g. Item 18: there are many different types of symptoms disturb you; about this item evaluation mainly on the basis of subjective description of patient, specific rating is as follows:

Score 0: no symptoms;

Score 1: there is one or two different kinds of symptoms exist, slightly feeling the pain;

Score 2: there are three different symptoms exist, painful feeling in gentle;

Score 3: there are three or above different symptoms exist, obviously feeling the pain;

Score 4: there are three different symptoms exist, severe pain sensation.

h. Item 19: you can't accept that your doctor told you have no disease;

The item refer to the "disease" is the concept of the public thinks that the existing pathological damage, and the so-called "organic disease", specific rating is as follows:

Level 0: fully believe the doctor;

Level 1: concern about condition , dispels concerns after the doctor told;

Level 2: still with faint worries, require further examination, although the doctor told no medical problem;

Level 3: still worried about the disease and want to be checked out after the doctor told no medical problem, and auxiliary examination is normal;

Level 4: do not believe that it is normal, although the doctor told no medical problem, and auxiliary examination is normal.

i. Item 26: difficulty falling asleep; assess the problems on the basis of two aspects: The current international industry recognized standards for the sleep difficulties that is to go to bed to sleep time after more than 30 minutes; And difficulty sleeping standard of this scale setting is "1 hour", that is to say, the symptoms were evaluated by the objective standard at least more than 30 minutes, two kinds of expression is not a contradiction. In addition, it is worth noting that the assessment of the item of the patient's subjective experience and description focuses on the specific time, if patients insist they have trouble falling asleep, it should be recorded as symptoms of the rating is based on the frequency and impact on himself, and ignores the time. Specific rating is as follows:

Score 0: no symptoms;

Score 1: It takes about one hour to fall asleep, once or twice within two weeks;

Score 2: It takes more than one hour to fall asleep, once or twice within one week;

Score 3: It takes more than one hour to fall asleep, more than 3 times within one week;

Score 4: unable to sleep completely, or even can't fall asleep all night, almost every day within one week.

j. Item 27: shallow sleep; the meaning of the "shallow sleep" and specific criteria as shown in the following:

Score 0: no such symptoms;

Score 1: basically know what happened around after sleeping, but did not wake up fully;

Score 2: know all the things happening around after sleeping, and easy to wake up, sleep again after waking up;

Score 3: a slight sound can be awakened himself, and then can fall asleep again;

Score 4: deficiency of sleep feeling even woke up by a slight ring and hard to fall asleep.

k. Item 28: early awakening; specific rating is as follows:

Score 0: no symptoms;

Score 1: wake up earlier for an hour than usual, once or twice within two weeks;

Score 2: wake up earlier for an hour than usual, about twice within one week;

Score 3: wake up earlier for more than an hour than usual, and more than three times within one week;

Score 4: wake up earlier for more than an hour than usual, almost every day within this week.

l. Item 29: easily tired after waking; here say "symptoms" refers to all the negative experiences, including emotions and all kinds of somatic symptoms. The specific standard is:

Score 0: no symptoms;

Score 1: find a little weak and tired after waking up, but the daily life cannot be affected;

Score 2: find weak and tired after waking up, daytime naps, and the daily life becomes a little difficult;

Score 3: find obvious weak and tired after waking up, and the daily life significantly be affected;

Score 4: find serious weak and tired after waking up, and it affected the daily life seriously.

m. Item 30: dreaminess; the item focuses on an individual's negative experience to dream. During sleep studies have shown that human sleep, dreams mainly appear in the quick eye movement (REM) sleep stages, and in adulthood REM sleep make up about a third of the total sleep time or fourth of the total sleep, that is to say, dream in the sleep is a normal situation. Some people describe their "dreaming" all night from sleep physiology perspective is impossible, whereas people describe their "all night without dreams" understanding of sleep physiology is impossible. As a result, this item is mainly of dreams by individual assessment negative experience, though if the critics responded to your dream experience and memory, but not of the negative experiences of dreams, shall be deemed to have the symptoms. In dreams in certain patients with negative experience, according to the following criteria to evaluate the degree of the patients:

Score 0: no symptoms;

Score 1: can feel several dreams after falling sleep, content is mostly clearly, but no big impact on the mood;

Score 2: have a series of dreams after falling sleep, content was clearly, and more for intense horrible dreams, no significant impact on the mood after waking;

Score 3: feeling dreaming the whole night, contents were more for intense and horrible, slightly affected the mood after waking;

Score 4: feeling dreaming the whole night, all contents were intense and horrible, and tension cannot be calm for a long time after waking.

n. Item 31: frequent micturition; it is also a score base on the subjective experience, with a specific number of relations is not big, but is closely related to individual experience of the phenomenon. Specific rating is as follows:

Score 0: no symptoms;

Score 1: be aware of the number of micturition slightly increasing, but it is still acceptable;

Score 2: be aware of the number of micturition increasing, feeling uneasy;

Score 3: be aware of the number of micturition increasing obviously, and want again after urinating, negative impact on some daily life;

Score 4: be aware of the number of micturition increasing seriously, feel urine was not solved usually, and make a serious impact on daily life.

o. Item 32: without any power sense; "no power" mainly meaning "helpless" situation, so it is "energy" as a basis for assessing the situation, and "no desire" is not included. Specific rating is as follows:

Score 0: no symptoms;

Score 1: feeling energy a little worse, but it does not influence the daily life and work;

Score 2: feeling lack of energy slightly, activitiess becomes slow, difficult to work, can maintain daily life basically;

Score 3: feeling lack of energy obviously, activitiess becomes slow, too hard to finish the work, and more difficult for daily life;

Score 4: feeling lack of energy seriously, activities become slow obviously, completely unable to do work or maintain the daily lives.

p. Item 33: loss of libido; specific grade see the following. Worthy of note is that no matter what, as long as the following conditions shall be according to the following standard scoring.

Score 0: no symptoms;

Score 1: no request for sex, but can complete sex with spouse;

Score 2: no request for sex, and the spouse's sexual demands can't be happy to cooperate;

Score 3: no request for sex, no response to sex requirement of spouses;

Score 4: no request for sex completely, as far as possible to avoid a spouse's sexual requirements;

q. **Item 38**: ulcer; scoring standards can be found in ulcers and their impact on individual criteria.

Score 0: no symptoms;

Score 1: once oral ulcer or gastric ulcer occurred within two weeks, with light pain;

Score 2: once or twice oral ulcer or gastric ulcer occurred within one week, with general pain;

Score 3: there are several times episodes of the ulcer pain occurred within one week, with serious pain;

Score 4: persistent ulcers and cause recurrent sever pain.

r. **Item 39**: no interest to do something(not with energy): the item with the item 32 the damage done by "no power" seems to be similar, but the pathological psychological mechanism is difference. If the item 32 "overwhelmed", referred to in this item is "strong uninterntionally" or "not weakness". Namely the item emphasizes evaluation behavior "motivation", or an individual desire, and the item 32 refers to as an executive motivation with conditions. In some actual cases, both exist at the same time, and in some cases, there is only one of them is often appeared in former underpowered. So when asking patients and specific rating differences should be paid attention to.

Score 0: no symptoms;

Score 1: be a little interesting in the new things, but is interesting in past favorite ;

Score 2: be a little interesting in the new things and is less interesting in past favorite;

Score 3: not interesting in new things and past favorite.

Score 4: server not interesting in new things and past favorite.

s. Item 48: more sensitive to pain than others; this is also a requirement by the critics make a subjective judgment problem, patients make evaluation is based on the compare myself with the surrounding people, while also contains your situation compared to their normal condition.

Score 0: No such circumstances;

Score 1: be sensitive to body's change, and sometimes concerns faintly to health;

Score 2: be sensitive to body's change, often worry about health, but the attention can be transferred;

Score 3: be sensitive body's change, worry about health excessively, require to control hardly, otherwise the attention can be transferred more difficultly;

Score 4: be extremely sensitive to body's change, and extremely worry about health, the attention cannot be transferred.

t. Item 49: experiencing physical symptoms are diversity and variability; specific rating is as follows:

Score 0: symptoms are single and fixed, no variability or diversity;

Score 1: it's not fixed of location for symptoms, the nature of the pain is similar, and caused slightly pain;

Score 2: it's not fixed of location for symptoms, the nature of the pain is , multiple, and caused some pain;

Score 3: it's not fixed of location for symptoms, the nature of the pain is, multitudinous, and caused heavily pain;

Score 4: it's not fixed of location for symptoms, the nature of the pain is, multitudinous, caused severe pain.

u. Item 50: you are more worried about health than most people; specific rating is as follows:

Score 0: no symptoms;

Score 1: the same degree of injury, you react to pain slightly sensitive than others;

Score 2: the same degree of injury, you react to pain slightly heavier than the others, and with slightly emotional reactions;

Score 3: the same degree of injury, you react to pain significantly more serious than others, and with obviously emotional reactions.

Score 4: the same degree of injury, you react to pain obviously serious than others, and the emotional reactions are particularly evident.

v. Item 51: if a disease brought to your attention, such as by radio, television, newspapers or someone you know, you worry about developing the disease, or link their discomfort associated with it; specific rating is as follows:

Score 0: no worries;

Score 1: faintly worry for two weeks, but can dispel this idea quickly;

Score 2: concerns about twice frequency one week, should find all kinds of information to dispel the idea;

Score 3: frequently concern more than three times a week or once a day, it is difficult to divert attention; although a lot of information about the sypmtoms he appear, but it difficult to convince myself;

Score 4: concentrate on symptoms actively, firmly believe in suffering from the disease, and the fears appear several times a day, all attention focused on this, cannot give up this idea in various ways.

4. Specified of peer assessment of the four items

Each of the following are peer assessments, specific score is based on each principle doctors performed as described.

Item 52: medical laboratory examination; specific rating is as follows:

Score 0: all auxiliary examinations have no positive finding;

Score 1: routine examinations have positive findings, such as biochemistry routine, blood routine, urine and stool routine, etc;

Score 2: auxiliary examinations have positive findings, but only as a reference for the diagnosis of disease;

Score 3: auxiliary examinations which are not the gold standard for diagnosis of the disease have positive findings, such as imaging (MRI, CT, etc.), ECG, EMG, ultrasound, and can be used as a basis for diagnosis of the disease;

Score 4: auxiliary examinations which are the gold standard for diagnosis of disease have positive findings, such as pathology, bacterial culture, etc.

Notes: Auxiliary examinations include laboratory examination, ECG, EEG, EMG, lung function, X-ray, ultrasound, endoscopy, radionuclide examination, etc. There are hundreds of examinations like these, each roles in disease diagnosis are different, meanwhile, they can be used as a reference for a different ratings. For example, the same laboratory examinations, some of these can only be taken as a reference, while others are used as a diagnostic basis. Every doctor gives a score judging by the above rating project and the role of auxiliary examination based on doctor's judgment in the diagnosis of disease in the specific disease judgment.

Item 53: diseases with definite diagnosis; specific rating is as follows:

Score 0: there is no definite diagnosis of the disease;

Score 1: there is one kind of diagnosis of the disease within the past three months;

Score 2 : there are two kind of diagnosis of the disease within the past three months;

Score 3: there are three kind of diagnosis of the disease within the past three months;

Score 4: there are four kind of diagnosis of the disease within the past three months;

Item 54: positive signs from doctors' examinations; specific rating is as follows:

Score 0: no positive signs;

Score 1: there are positive signs, but it has no significant contact with medical history description;

Score 2: there are positive signs, which is consistent with medical history, but the symptoms are mild and it doesn't be considered as a reference for the diagnosis of disease;

Score 3: there are positive signs, which is consistent with medical history, and it can be used as reference for the diagnosis of disease;

Score 4: there are positive signs, which is consistent with medical history, and it can be used as a basis for the diagnosis of disease.

Item 55: visible damage; specific rating is as follows:

Score 0: no visible damage;

Score 1: some slight visible damage exist with small-scale, mild sensory symptoms in patients;

Score 2: some significant visible damage exists with small-scale, severe sensory symptoms in patients;

Score 3: some significant visible damage exists with large range, and the patient feels very serious. It can offer some medical treatment some days;

Score 4: there is some serious visible damage, and aggressive medical treatment needs to be done as soon as possible.

5. The scale interpretation of results

A. Score analysis

a. Total scores reflect the severity of the disease. The so-called "severity" mainly refers to the pain of patients and the effects of daily life for patients. The condition is more sever and the score is higher.

b. The gap of the total score before and after treatment reflect the evolution of the disease, which is a main purpose of setting total score.

c. In terms of the specific patients, reduction rate can be used to determine efficacy assessment, reduction rate = (total score before treatment – total score after treatment)/total score before treatment. It is generally believed that reduction rate≥50% shows efficacy remarkable, ≥25% is valid.

B. Analysis of individual score

a. Individual score reflects the specific symptom distribution: Symptoms Rating Scale is a tool of assessing his clinical symptoms and the scale of the individual score to reflect the distribution of specific clinical symptoms. The single points of the scale not only can reflect the distribution of the specific clinical symptoms types, but also can get some specific patient's the most outstanding results of what kind of somatic symptoms. According to this result, provide an important basis for formulating treatment plan. For example, irritability somatic symptoms were to anti-anxiety-based treatment, inhibitory somatic symptoms were to anti-depression-based treatment, cognitive somatic symptoms were to typical antipsychotics to improve cognition based treatment and so on.

b. Individual score reflect therapeutic effect of target symptoms: changes of scores before and after treatment in scale also can reflect the status of each target to improve symptoms. We can take respectively t-test analysis towards the changes of individual points before and after treatment, so that it can show the treatment effect of target symptoms through the changes of individual points.

C. Factor analysis and outline map

a. Computing factor scores: factor scores = composition of the individual factor scores / composition of the number of the factors of the project.

b. The treatment results of the target symptom clusters is reflected through analysis of factors: One of the main purposes of symptom rating scales is used for efficacy evaluation, yet through factor molecules, it can reflects the results of target symptoms treatment group.

c. Outline map: outline diagram before and after treatment.

The significance of the profile is to understand the specific patient's overall situation so that it can provide a basis for individualized treatment for each individual patient. For example, A and B of two patients with the highest scoring factors are "irritable somatic symptoms", A with sub-high factor is "cognitive somatic symptoms", while B with sub-high factor is "imaginary symptoms". At this time, A treatment regimen should be anti anxiety drugs + atypical antipsychotic drugs, and B treatment programs should be anti anxiety drugs + comprehensive treatment (including psychological counseling, symptomatic treatment, *etc.*). For example, A patient was identified as "biological somatic symptoms", showed that the pathological damage plays an important role in the generation of negative experience. But as expressed in the first chapter of the consensus point of view, since the somatic symptoms are "unpleasant subjective feeling", then any somatic symptoms should be related to individual cognition, emotion, personality and other psychological factors. That's why the same damage in different individuals have different reasons of negative experiences in different degrees and even different forms. This kind of patients with somatic symptoms of physical and psychological treatment are based mainly the profile of the scale, especially the sub-high factor. For example, The highest score of a patient is "biological somatic symptoms", and the sub-high factor is "irritable somatic symptoms". At this time, the treatment of somatic symptoms of the patient should be: treatment of pathological damage + anti-anxiety treatment.

D. Factor distribution

In the four clusters of physical symptoms, Emotional somatic symptoms can be divided into Suppression somatic symptoms and irritation somatic symptoms, so the scale can be divided into five factors.

Suppression somatic symptoms(a): **4, 5, 28, 29, 32, 33, 34, 36, 37, 39, 41, 47**.

b. Irritation somatic symptoms (b): 2, 3, 9, 26, 27, 30, 31, 35, 38, 40, 42, 43, 45, **46**.

c. Biological somatic symptoms(c): **52, 53, 54, 55, 8**.

d. Imagine somatic symptoms (d): **15, 16, 17, 18, 19, 23, 48, 49, 50, 51**.

e. Cognitive somatic symptoms (e): **1, 6, 7, 10, 11, 12, 13, 14, 20, 21, 22, 24, 25, 44**.

E. Calculation method

a. Factor scores: factor score = sum of each item of the factor / item number. For example: Computational Biology somatic symptoms score = sum of scores of projects 3, 4, 6, 10, 12 / 5 (five items).

b. Total: 55 items total score is symptom score.

6. Interpretation of results

a. The higher scores indicate the more severe symptoms.

b. Significance of factor: The highest score of a factor reveals a patient's the main properties of somatic symptoms, but also provides a direction of treatment programs.

c. Significance of the scale profile: Just like the role of personality rating scale, the profile of the scale can be shown the whole picture of somatic symptoms appeared in the patients, but also providing a reference for the treatment of individual. That is , providing an important reference for the development of a comprehensive treatment plan for a patient, that is, providing an important reference for the "treatment of precision".

d. Through the measurement of the scale before and after treatment, through the total score or calculation of the reduction rate of a factor, to provide basis for evaluation and research of therapeutic effect.

e. There are a lot of items in the scale, and the problems need to be further accurate and standardized. At the same time, in the first chapter, the possible existence of "rhythmic symptoms" has not been passed through the test, obtaining relevant evidence and other issues need to be improved in the revision.

(Fanmin Zeng)

Chapter 3　Multi-center on-site investigation of WCPA-SSCS(revised-1) under the theoretical framework of psychosomatic medicine

Section 1　A brief introduction to the method

A. overview

Based on previous work, we verified the hypothesis of somatic symptom classification theory under the concept of psychosomatic medicine with clinical data from a psychometric angle, and developed the assesement tool WCPA Somatic Symptom Classification Scale(second edition) (WCPA-SSCS). Furthermore, the project group had conducted a empirical research on this hypothesis. The final conclusion was that the somatic symptom classification theory hypothesis was tenable, and WCPA-SSCS(R-1) had good reliability and validity to be used as a measurement tool for somatic symptoms.

Based on this, a multi-center on-site investigation was carried out in comprehensive hospitals and psychiatric hospitals nationwide using WCPA-SSCS(second edition) to explore the classification and treatment of somatic symptoms.

A total of 70 sites from 16 departments were included in this investigation. The 16 departments were neurology, cardiology, psychiatry, gastroenterology, psychosomatic medicine, psychology, pain, sleep center, rehabilitation, geriatrics, spleen and stomach (traditional chinese medicine), and andrology (Table 3-1-1). All investigators in each site received training about the study and clearly understood the theory hypoth-

esis, classification tool WCPA-SSCS(R-1), study protocal and method of
operation. The investigation lasted 6 months.

Table 3-1-1   Department distribution information

Department	Percentage(%)
Neurology	32.2
Gastroenterology	17.3
Psychosomatic medicine	17.3
Pain	5.7
Psychiatry	5.1
Psychology	4.9
Andrology	3.0
Cardiology	3.7
Sleep center	3.0
Rehabilitation	1.4
Spleen and stomach	1.0
Geriatrics	1.0
Otolaryngology	0.4
General family medicine	2.0
Dermatology	2.0
Total	100.0

B. The flow chart of the study

The flow chart of this on-site investigation was showed as below.
The subjects who met inclusive and exclusive criteria were enrolled in
this on-site investigation and received recommended treatment according
to different somatic symptoms subtypes. Severity of somatic symptoms
and endocrine indexes were assessed at baseline, 4 weeks and 12 weeks.

The aims of this on-site investigation were: i) further verify somatic
symptoms classification hypothesis in a larger scope; ii) verify the reliability and feasibility of WCPA-SSCS (second edition) in a larger scope;

iii) to explore the efficacy of recommended treatment regimens according to subtypes of somatic symptoms to further verify the tenability of somatic symptoms classification hypothesis and provide evidence for somatic symptoms treatment; iv) To explore the treatment of the optimized treatment plan of all kinds of somatic symptoms.

C. Subjects

a. Inclusive criteria

i) 18 to 65 years old;

ii) Compliant of more than one somatic symptom regardless of existing diagnosis;

iii) The somatic symptoms resulted in the patient's concern, or great pain, or social function impairement.

b. Exclusive criteria

i) Acute infection, acute trauma, perioperative period, or acute phase of chronic diseases;

ii) In a critical condition or dying patients cannot participate in this study;

iii) Pregnancy or lactation women;

iv) Patients with substance abuse.

D. Method

a. The period of this on-site investigation was 12 weeks. Scale assessments and biological indexes examinations were done at 0, 4, 12 week. Used assessment tools were listed as follows(Table 3-1-2):

Table 3-1-2　List of assessment tools

Symptoms	Efficacy	Endocrine indexes
WCPA-SSCS	Clinical Global Impression, CGI	HPA axis
The Big Five Personality Inventory-Brief version	Treatment Emergent Symptom Scale, TESS	HPT axis
		Sex hormone
		OGTT

b. According to the scale of the assessment results of physical symptoms, respectively adopt the method of corresponding drugs or other corresponding treatment.

Section 2   Results of the on-site investigation

A. Demographic characteristics of enrolled subjects

Up to June 15, 2016, 2710 patients were screened and 2457 patients were enrolled (reclaimed rate was 90.67%). Clinical trial registration number for this study was ChiCTR - OCS - 14004632. Demographic information was as follows(Table 3-2-1):

Table 3-2-1   Demographic characteristics of enrolled subjects

Characteristics	Percentage(%)
Gender	
Male	35.2
Female	64.8
Age	
<20 years	2.0
20-29 years	8.6
30-39 years	15.8
40-49 years	27.7
50-59 years	28.6
60-65 years	17.3
Education	
Primary school or below	23.1
Junior high school	27.3
High school	23.0
Junior college	12.7
University	12.2
Graduate or above	1.8
Profession	
Employed	44.0
Retired	26.1
Unemployment	28.2

From the demographic data can at least see several notable characteristics: an a. somatic symptom in people with the low culture level is
obvious; b. somatic symptoms are concentrated in 40-60 years old in the
crowd; c. somatic symptoms are concentrated in the retired or unemployed population; d. group of women somatic symptoms than men; it is
worth to close attention to the characteristics of the above tips and future
research, especially for the low cultural level, female, and retired or unemployed, and so on the characteristics of attention and help to further
study on the comprehensive treatment of all kinds of somatic symptoms.

**B. Patient self-reported impacts on social function were pre-
sented in Table 3-2-2**

Table 3-2-2　Patient self-reported impacts on social function

Severity	Percentage(%)
No impact	8.5
Moderate impact	50.7
Severe impact	40.8

91.5% of the respondents reported their social function was impaired
by somatic symptoms which indicated that somatic discomfort was one of
the main reasons for patients to go to hospital.

**C. Patient self-reported concerning about somatic symptoms
were presented in Table 3-2-3**

Table 3-2-3　Patient self-reported concerning about somatic symptoms

Concern about somatic symptoms	Percentage(%)
No concern	3.3
Moderate concern	38.1
Highly concern	58.5

In this on-site investigation, 2457 subjects were enrolled (male: female, 35.2%: 64.8%), with mean age was 35.5 ±10.2 years old. The educational level in this sample was not high that mainly were junior high school or high school levels. Most of respondents were unemployed. 96.6% of the respondents reported their social function was impaired by somatic symptoms. The most common somatic symptoms was irritable somatic symptoms, followed by inhibitory somatic symptoms and cognitive somatic symptoms.

D. Distribution of somatic symptoms

According to the theroy of psychosomatic medicine, the distribution results of the 5 subtypes of somatic symptoms in this on-site investigation showed as follows (Table 3-2-4):

Table 3-2-4   Distribution of 5 types of somatic symptoms

Somatic symptoms type	Percentage(%)
Inhibitory somatic symptoms	41.9
Irritable somatic symptoms	21.9
Imaginative somatic symptoms	4.1
Biological somatic symptoms	11.2
Cognitive somatic symptoms	21.1

The results showed that the proportion of the emotional somatic symptoms was quite high. The highest subtype was inhibitory somatic symptoms. From the test results of 2014, ranking the first is "irritable somatic symptoms", the more realistic anxiety is a normal idea of individual basic emotions. And when combined with data from 2015-2016, present as a result of the "inhibitory somatic symptoms" ranked all the somatic symptoms of the first. As a field test of actual results, the authors show respect and publicly, but the reasons for this situation may have the following several aspects: a. participates in testers "inhibitory somatic symptoms" and "irritable somatic symptoms" recognition has not been fully agreed standards. b. the revised "scale" to distinguish between types of somatic symptoms has not sensitive and accurate enough. c. although according to common sense, irritable somatic symptoms should be more than the inhibitory somatic symptoms, but in view of the impact on the social function, the latter are clinic group than the former. d. the current test results is the real reflection of the actual situation. As for more accurate information, subject to further revision "scale" and the field test.

E. Results of scale factor analysis

According to the measurement data in this multi-center study, we verified the internal structure of WCPA-SSCS(second edition). The results were as follows:

a. Factor analysis of the appropriateness (Table 3-2-5)

Table 3-2-5 Appropriateness of factor analysis

Kaiser-Meyer-Olkin Measure of Sampling Adequacy		0.847
Bartletts Test of Sphericity	Approx. Chi-Square	6849.568
	df	1431
	Sig.	0.000

The results showed that the value of KMO was greater than 0.8, indicating the data was appropriate for factor analysis.

b. The cumulative variance contribution ratio of the factors (Table 3-2-6)

Table 3-2-6 the cumulative variance contribution ratio of the second-order factor

Component	Total	% of Variance	Cumulative (%)
1	7.181	39.395	39.395
2	3.479	7.217	46.612
3	3.190	6.912	53.524
4	2.163	6.895	60.419

The results showed that the cumulative variance contribution rate
was 60.419, indicating extraction of four common factors was desirable.
c. Scree plot Figure 3-2-1

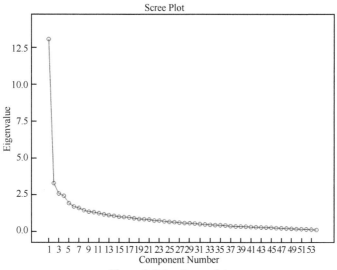

Figure 3-2-1   Scree plot

Factors were determined according to cumulative contribution rate
on the basis of characteristic value was greater than or equal to 1. Gravel
inspection results showed the numer of public factors was 4. The results
of this on-site investigation shows that the classification of the somatic
symptoms is reasonable; four kinds of classification of distribution has
certain clinical value.

F. Therapeutic effect evaluation

Based on the classification theory of somatic symptoms under psychosomatic medicine theroy, somatic symptoms could be divided into 5
subtypes. Recommended treatment regimens were made for each type of
somatic symptoms (specific recommended regimens can refer to section 4

in this chapter). According to the recommended treatment, all subjects received drug therapy combined with psychological therapy. Somatic symptoms were assessed at baseline, 1 month and 3 months after treatment which were efficacy indicators.

Therapeutic effect evaluation included two parts: one was WCPA-SSCS scores that reduction rate ⩾25% for effective and ⩾50% for significantly effective; and the other one was the change of endocrine indexes(Table 3-2-7).

Table 3-2-7   WCPA–SSCS scores at baseline, 4 weeks, and 12 weeks

	Baseline		4 weeks		12 weeks		F
	mean	sd	mean	sd	mean	sd	$P<0.01$
Total score	50.36	27.47	34.36	21.14	24.27	17.18	**
Inhibitory	51.41	27.99	35.57	21.35	24.16	16.22	**
Irritable	53.91	28.04	35.14	19.85	23.00	16.43	**
Biological	33.85	29.11	26.36	25.43	16.46	16.56	**
Imaginative	40.20	31.36	28.06	26.15	18.65	21.03	**
Cognitive	53.40	20.15	35.59	17.94	29.21	16.27	**

** note: treatment effect was significant that somatic symptoms significantly decreased at 1 month, 3 months after treatment.

By analyzing the proportion of ineffective, effective and significant effective of WCPA-SSCS at 1 month and 3 months, we found "effective" was highest at 1 month, with its proportion was 78.2%; "significantly effective" was highest at 3 months, with its proportion was 66.2%.

The change of endocrine indexes included:

i) TSH, FT_4, TT_3, and TT_4 significantly changed;

ii) FT_4 and TT_4 significantly changed in inhibitory somatic symptoms;

iii) FT_3 and ACTH significantly changed in irritable somatic symptoms;

iv) FT_4, TSH and TT_3 significantly changed in all kinds of somatic symptoms.

G. The personality characteristics of somatic symptoms

a. Introduction of the Big Five Personality Inventory [35]: namely the NEO personality inventory, was developed by the American psychologist Costa Costa and McRae McCrae in 1987 based on the theory of big five personality, and revised twice later. The Chinese version was revised by psychologist professor Zhang from Chinese academy of sciences. This questionnaire was a personality trait testing tool belonging to personality trait genre of personality theory. Five factors of personality included: extraversion, agreeableness, conscientiousness, emotional stability and openness to experience.

Extraversion: one side is extremely extroverted, and the other is extremely introverts. Extraverts enjoy interacting with people, are often perceived as full of energy, and are optimistic, friendly and confident. Introverts have lower social engagement than extraverts, which should not be interpreted as self-centeredness or lack of energy. Introverts prefer to implicative, autonomy and steady.

Agreeableness: the ones with higher scores are helpful, reliable, sympathetic and payed more attention on cooperation rather than competition; the ones with lower scores are hostility, suspicious and liked to fight for their own interests and beliefs.

Conscientiousness: is a tendency to show self-discipline and self-control. High scores on conscientiousness indicate a preference for planned, well organized behavior and are able to persevere. Lower scores indicate sloppy, easily fickle, and unreliable.

Emotional stability: higher scores indicate more easily upset on daily pressure. Lower scores indicate do well in self-adaptation and not easy to respond extremely.

Openness to experience: it is an opened attitude not only to communication, but also to experience. Higher score indicate nonconformists and thinking independently while lower scores indicate more traditional and used to familiar things than new things.

b. Results

Neuroticism (N): The lower scores, the greater stability of the emotions, and the higher scores, the less stability of the emotions. Typical low score was less than 20.4, and typical high score was greater than 38.8. In this study, the mean score was 31.46. It showed that patients with somatic symptoms had unstable emotion.

Extraversion (E): the higher scores, the more extraversion. Typical low score was less than 26, and typical high score was greater than 4. In this study the lowest was 10.31, and the highest was 43.1. It showed that patients with somatic symptoms were at both extremes of extraversion.

Openness to experience (O): the higher scores, the more openness. Typical low score was less than 32, and typical high score was greater than 47. In this study the lowest was 8.95, and the highest was 28.89. It showed that patients with somatic symptoms were not openness.

Agreeableness (A): the higher score, the more easygoing personality. Typical low score was less than 30, and typical high score was greater than 48. In this study the lowest was 9.25, and the highest was 30.74. It showed that patients with somatic symptoms were not easygoing.

Conscientiousness (C): the higher score, the stronger responsibility. Typical low score was less than 36, and typical high score was greater than 44. In this study the lowest was 11.10, and the highest is 34.34. It showed that patients with somatic symptoms were not stronger responsibility.

Section 3   The interpretation of on-site investigation result

Personality refers to the mental profile of a person in such aspects as characteristic, temperament and competence, the individual's attitude to reality and environment and habits of behavior. Personality traits and character flaw are the main factors for susceptibility to psychosomatic disease, and the basis and cause of psychosomatic disease. For example, a person with adequate personality is less susceptible to the influence of major life event; on the other side, the person will be more susceptible to the influence of the major life events, or there might be occurrence of mental or physical diseases. This study found that the in the enrolled patients with somatic symptoms, the personality characteristics included emotional instability, bipolar, not easy-going, introvert, and less responsible. These factors are bases for psychosomatic disease. Fukud *et al* used temperament and personality questionnaire investigated 211 cases of chronic fatigue syndrome patients and 90 normal subjects in the personality differences, and the results found that patients with chronic fatigue syndrome showed more neurotic tendencies.

This study found that the neurotic personality traits were more significant in people with somatic symptoms. The research results and the previous research results obtained are consistent. Neuroticism is one of the core factors of personality traits, which reflects the individual risk perception and experiences degree of outside chaos. The higher personality trait scores, the more intense and frequent negative emotions reported, the effected may experience low self-confident, more stress, and anxiety. The study found that exaggerating somatic symptoms is also one of the basic characteristics of neurotic personality. Somatic symptoms score as the dependent variable research has shown that neuroticism was significantly positively correlated to personality and somatic symptoms.

In a multi-center clinical study of clinical classification of somatic symptoms, different study protocols were recommended for different somatic symptoms. The field test results indicated the treatment effect is marked. We, on the other hand, studied the neuroendocrine indicators of somatic symptoms, and found that after 1 month, 3 months neuroendocrine indicators had a tend to be greatly increased, which had significant differences from the baseline, reaching to the statistical significance level ($p < 0.05$, $p < 0.01$). Study results showed that the interpretation of clinical symptoms from the perspective of psychosomatic medicine and the classification into four large dimensions are scientific and reasonable.

Of all the 2475 patients enrolled, the biological somatic symptoms were 4.1% in the all group. The results also provide us thinking: whether there are inevitability changes between somatic symptoms and biological symptoms? According to the logic reason enough to law, in the uncertain pathological damage is a connection between somatic symptoms and clinical in most cases, the overall disease treatment should include three dimensions, namely the etiological treatment dimension, pathology, physiology and pathology of psychological dimension and semeiology dimension treatment. In treatment of angina pectoris , for example, the cause shall be the diversified factors, including genetic factors, personality factors and environmental factors; Its pathophysiological mechanism for coronary artery disease; Its symptoms are irritable body symptoms. So the treatment should include: i) for etiological treatment, due to the diversity of pathogenic factors, perhaps for many cases, the treatment is difficult to truly complete; ii) pathological physiology treatment, namely, no matter use what means, to improve the treatment of coronary artery is the main goal. iii) symptomatic treatment for symptomatic treatment of the situation are mainly through the use of powerful anti-anxiety drugs to reduce or eliminate the pain. The idea of "three dimensions" treatment is the concrete embodiment of psychosomatic development theory, and need further validation and share in this concept, in order to get more recognition of clinical workers.

From the point of the field test results, we tend to be no consistency between them, and to promote the understanding and exploring of somatic symptoms should hold an open attitude, there is no connection between the symptoms and damage, somatic symptoms associated with personality traits more. However, from the perspective of psychosomatic medicine, the handling of somatic symptoms at the same time shall be from two aspects: one is the separate treatment of pathological symptoms; and the second is to the treat somatic symptoms separately. In the follow-up study, the idea that somatic symptoms as the third clinical pathological character shall be strengthened.

Through clinical multi-center field test data, we once again conducted confirmatory analysis of the WCPA somatic symptom classification scale, the results proved once again that scientificity and rationality of the interpretation of somatic symptoms under the framework of psychosomatic medicine theory, showing that the measuring tool has good reliability and validity, which can be used in clinical practice. The somatic symptoms classification and practice can be an important basis for identification and treatment of somatic symptom. See chapter 4 for the treatment.

(Fanmin Zeng)

Chapter 4   Under the framework of the psychosomatic medicine theory classification treatment of somatic symptoms: a multilateral field test results-summary

Section 1   Optimization of treatment recommendations

First, about the idea of optimization treatment recommendations

Mentioned earlier, according to the concept of psychosomatic medicine somatic symptom types are divided into emotional somatic symptoms (irritation symptoms and inhibitory somatic symptoms), cognitive somatic symptom, imaginative somatic symptoms, and biological somatic symptoms. In the third chapter, have described the WCPA somatic symptom classification scale of testing(second edition), analysis and prove the existence of psychosomatic disorder classification. Described in this chapter is mainly about the classification of the symptoms of drug treatment.

The recommended optimization of the treatment scheme is based on the theory of psychosomatic medicine composition of different types of somatic symptoms resolve give corresponding treatment respectively. As for irritable somatic symptoms with anti-anxiety treatment; For the use of antidepressant methods in inhibitory somatic symptom treatment; The cognitive somatic symptoms in order to improve cognitive and adjust the mood as the treatment goal; For imaginative somatic symptoms, to improve the cognitive, planning life, adjust the mood, to establish a good interpersonal relationship and accelerate the development of his personality as the comprehensive treatment goal, which in addition to the recommended drug treatment, also includes emphasis on the role of psychological guidance for the treatment of such symptoms; The author thinks that the biological somatic symptoms, since is the essence of the somatic symptoms "unpleasant subjective feeling", by this reasoning, any physical symptoms associated with psychological factors. For the analysis of the biological body symptoms should be admitted that the role of pathological damage in produce symptoms, pathological damage at the same time should be lined factors separately analyze the individual's physical symptoms to determine the individualized treatment goals of this kind of physical symptoms, such as improving cognition and adjust the mood, that is to say, on the basis of pathological damage treatment for patients at the same time on the psychosomatic comprehensive treatment of the symptoms.

Second, according to the specific recommendations of all kinds of symptoms of treatment

A. Recommendations for the treatment of irritable somatic symptoms

Had mentioned in the previous section the "consensus", as defined by the irritable somatic symptoms for organ dysfunction is a basic feature of symptoms, such as intestinal irritability syndrome, pain, because this kind of symptom reflects the organs increased alertness, so anti-anxiety treatment should be the basic principles for the treatment of such symptoms. In addition, the pathological anxiety produce abnormal cognitive, so treat pathological anxiety should include experience, cognitive, and suit the three dimensions. Based on the above considerations, the basic principles of treatment of irritable somatic symptoms should include anti-anxiety, improved cognition and experience. According to the front of the train of thought, irritable body symptom treatment recommendations are as follows:

a. SSRI drugs (selective serotonin reuptake inhibitors) + atypical anti-psychotics, medium and long half-life of benzodiazepines drugs scheme: this project for irritable somatic symptoms in the recommended SSRI drugs mainly includes paroxetine, sertraline and escitalopram citalopram and citalopram; Based on the efficacy, safety and clinical physicians, par-ticularly is a mental habit of specialist clinicians use of psychotropic drugs, recommended in the project of atypical antipsychotics mainly in-cludes the olanzapine and quetiapine flat; Recommended in the project of the medium and long-term benzodiazepines drugs mainly alprazolam and clonazepam.

b. SSRI drugs + atypical antipsychotics, non benzodiazepines anti-anxiety drug solution: this scenario the recommended specific SSRI drugs and atypical antipsychotics and plan a is the same, and for those main irritable somatic symptoms as chief complaint but no patients with sleep disorders, this recommendation will be replaced benzodiazepines drugs than the non-benzodiazepines drugs. Specific recommendations of drugs is the main tandospirone. In clinical practice, clinicians can also use other drugs in the drug.

c. SNRI drugs + atypical antipsychotics, medium and long half-life of benzodiazepines drugs + tiapride will benefit plan: in this scenario, the recommended specific SSRI drugs, atypical antipsychotics and the me-dium and long half-life benzodiazepines drugs are the same as the front, and recommend tiapride is especially for patients with pain symptoms.

d. Flupentixol and melitracen tablets + medium and long half-life benzo-diazepines drugs: Flupentixol and melitracen tablets is a compound prep-aration including flupentixol and melitracen, the former is the first gener-ation antipsychotics, the latter for the tricyclic antidepressants, so choose the drug's purpose is to improve the experience of anxiety and cognitive, and benzodiazepines drugs is added to strengthen the effect of improving the effects of sleep and early anti-anxiety.

e. Proprietary chinese medicine scheme: the current domestic numerous for mood disorders of proprietary chinese medicine, but the results of the study isn't consistent. Considering the safety of the drug, also considering the cultural background of chinese patients and further in the natural en-vironment of proprietary chinese medicine clinical curative effect of ob-servation, in the field test is recommended with recent studies prove that focus allow for effective wuling capsule and shugan jieyu capsule as a proprietary chinese medicine for the treatment of irritable somatic symp-toms. Clinicians can use alone, and on the basis of large sample to sum-marize the curative effect, also can according to the actual situation of patients, the above recommended as the main treatment, and the two drugs as auxiliary drug use.

B. Recommendations for the treatment of inhibitory somatic symptoms

Weak body symptom is reflected in this consensus means of organ function or weakening of symptoms, such as abdominal distension, ano-rexia, functional dyspepsia syndrome. At the same time, this consensus assumes that the inhibitory body symptoms is pathological depression body, therefore antidepressant treatment become the main target for the treatment of such symptoms. In addition, the produce of pathological de-pression first based on distorted cognition (not give meaning to life), followed by the depressed state of mind, then there is chaos in the biological rhythm, so treatment of pathological depression should include improve the cognitive dimensions, improve the experience and adjusting rhythm treatment. Similarly, since the inhibitory somatic symptoms as a treatment, pathological depression in the optimal treatment is recommended, also based on the previously mentioned three dimensions.

a. SNRI drugs (selective serotonin and norepinephrine reuptake inhibitor) + atypical antipsychotics, medium and long half-life benzodiazepines drug solution: because of the dual role of SNRI drugs currently in psychiatric profession is regarded as main antidepressants. In the scenario the recommended specific drugs including venlafaxine and duloxetine, venlafaxine, for example, in the case of a 150 mg daily volume, its effect is equivalent to an SSRI drugs, which have the effect of serotonin reuptake inhibitors, the dose of 225 mg or more, on the central nervous system of play serotonin and norepinephrine reuptake inhibition effect, and the daily dose of 300 mg or more, then in addition to play serotonin and norepinephrine reuptake inhibition, still can effect the dopamine system of the central nervous system. So these drugs can not only improve the feelings of depression, and can improve depression cognitive, that is what will be the class as the main causes of antidepressant drug, is the basis of this consensus assumes that inhibitory somatic symptoms pathological depression, that inhibitory somatic symptoms of depression disorder's body form, therefore recommend such drugs for the treatment of inhibiting the body symptoms mainly drugs; Recommended in the scheme of the atypical antipsychotics remains for the olanzapine and quetiapine. In the recommended scheme is on the use of atypical antipsychotics, reason and the treatment of irritable body symptoms are the same, namely to strengthen to improve the patient's perception, and for the treatment of pathological depression, improve cognition is more important and necessary; And the recommended, medium and long half-life of benzodiazepines drugs as part of the package is the purpose of improving patient treatment early feelings and sleep problems, specific drugs and treatment is the same irritable somatic symptoms.

b. SSRI drugs + atypical antipsychotics, medium and long half-life benzodiazepines drugs: choice of atypical antipsychotics and benzodiazepines drugs recommended reasons and specific drugs and the first solution is the same, go here. This plan referred to in the SSRI drugs mainly fluoxetine.Previous research and clinical practice showed that fluoxetine can be applied to the thyroid gland axis, and improve individual's lack of motivation, thus it is recommended to use in the treatment of inhibiting the body symptoms.

c. SNRI drugs/SSRI drugs + mood stabilizers, atypical antipsychotics plan: in the recommended scheme is chosen SNRI drugs, SSRI drugs, and the reason of atypical antipsychotics and concrete suggestions to use drugs is the same as the second scheme. Recommend the use of mood stabilizers reason lies in the psychiatric profession think pathological depression in recent years were part of the dysrhythmia, and studies have shown that mood stabilizer main therapy effect is stable biological rhythms, such as emotional rhythm. Now that the consensus assumes that inhibitory body form, physical symptom is the pathological depression is recommended to use mood stabilizer as part of the treatment of inhibiting the body symptoms salience. The recommended in the field test of mood stabilizers of specific drugs including lamotrigine and sodium valproate. Lithium carbonate for psychiatric profession recognized has exact curative effect of mood stabilizers, but considering the safety of psychiatric medicine specialist clinicians the familiarity of the drug and the acceptance of the psychiatric patients on the drug, such as the specific circumstances, therefore, in this scenario is not recommended directly, but the spirit of the familiar with the drug specialist according to the specific circumstances of patients with the drug into the treatment plan.

d. About using other SSRI drugs as the core of combination plan: according to reports in the literature in addition to the fluoxetine, the rest of the SSRI medications have antidepressant effect, although not specifically recommended, therefore, in clinical field test in natural conditions, clinicians, according to the actual situation of patients using SSRI drugs other than the fluoxetine and as the core of combination regimen for inhibiting the body symptoms accepted by the field test.

e. Proprietary Chinese medicine combination scheme: see the treatment of irritable somatic symptoms.

C. Recommendations for the treatment of cognitive somatic symptoms

About cognitive somatic symptoms please refer to the concept of the first chapter of the related content. The need to further illustrate the problem is that in the clinical practice of cognitive somatic symptoms include two aspects, one is refers to the patients with negative interpretation of body information, the concept of this idea and psychiatric specialist hypochondriacal very close, and the goal of treatment is mainly to improve the patient's cognitive; the other is in line with the illusion defined body symptoms, the characteristics of this kind of symptom is: ①comply with the illusion of definition, namely no objective stimulation on sensory organs from sensory organs direct access to the unreal feeling; ②parts relatively fixed; ③description is clear. For the treatment of this kind of situation goals include to improve cognitive and adjust the negative experience. According to the goal of treatment for cognitive somatic symptoms of recommendation consists of the following conditions.

a. Separate with atypical antipsychotics: considering the spiritual practitioner drug habit, for patients who are familiar with the situation of the psychotropic drugs and avoid extrapyramidal reactions, the scheme firstly recommended olanzapine as a preferred drug, moreover the clinician can also according to the goal of treatment and their habit of psychotropic drugs, and drug experience as like quetiapine flat or other atypical anti-psychotics as main treatment drugs.

b. Flupentixol and melitracen Tablets scheme: the drug is a tricyclic anti-depressants and first-generation antipsychotic drugs in line with the prep-aration, the cognitive physical symptoms recommend this medicine is the purpose of improving the cognition and bad experience.

c. Atypical antipsychotics + SSRI drugs: specific atypical antipsychotics are still mainly recommend the olanzapine and quetiapine flat, and spe-cific SSRI drugs still recommend paroxetine, sertraline and escitalopram citalopram and citalopram. Still based on the purpose of the scheme com-bination treatment goals for the cognitive body symptoms, namely to im-prove cognitive and eliminate bad experience.

D. Recommendations for the treatment of imaginative somatic symptoms

About the connotation of the concept of imaginative somatic symp-toms, please see the first chapter. Imaginative somatic symptoms are based on hints or self-talk cases produced by the type of symptoms.The symptoms than other classes of a more complex pathological physiologi-cal and pathological psychological root, specifically speaking, this kind of symptom and individual quality, early life of the natural and humanistic environment, personality traits, interpersonal relationship, the education background, life events and the current emotional state, and many other factors related.Treatment of these symptoms should be more personal-ized, therefore, need to be determined to evaluate treatment of individuals with specific treatment of specific individuals of the current and long-term goals, adopted by the drug treatment according to the specific

· 134 · Consensus for Psychosomatic Classification, Diagnosis and Treatment
of Somatic Symptoms

treatment of the identified target see face three kinds of symptoms before the recommended treatment plan. In addition, special is worth questioning for the treatment of this kind of symptom, highlighted the role of psychological counselling more, because the treatment for this kind of symptom is more personalized features, put forward in this unfavorable relatively unified psychological intervention or counseling model. About the treatment regularity of this kind of problem, particularly in terms of psychological counseling the regularity of the accumulation of information needs to be treated case.

E. Recommendations for the treatment of biological somatic symptoms

The concept of biological body symptom still see relevant contents of the first chapter, on the need to further illustrate the so-called biological physical symptoms mainly refers to the individual for evidence of pathological damage, and also no clear evidence that the existing of the pathological damage and there is no connection between the symptoms of the condition. Since this consensus is the basic idea of somatic symptoms is the "unpleasant subjective feeling", feel or experience is an important psychological function, so any physical symptoms associated with psychological factors. Based on this idea, the principle is in the treatment of biological body symptoms in the treatment of pathological damage at the same time, according to the specific psychological assessment of patients to determine the target of comprehensive treatment of the patients, such as "improve cognition", "adjust mood", "strengthen the psychological motivation", *etc.*, which is for the treatment of this kind of symptom is the basic principle of physical and mental development. And about the specific recommendations, can see the first few classes symptom treatment recommendations. Under natural conditions for such symptoms in clinical field test purpose is to hope to prove that any physical symptoms and psychological factors related to the concept and prove the somatic symptoms rather than as a stand-alone treatment dimension is attached to the necessity of the "disease".

Third, about the recommended solutions to problems

a. Above all recommended scheme is only a hint, recommended scheme is put forward from literature, case analysis, some clinicians' medical experience, which reference for clinicians. Without limiting the recommended regimen clinicians under the condition of natural medicine.The results of field test statistics will be subject to the actual clinical medication information.

b. With the recommended scheme of all drugs are listed, so relevant information about the various drug such as mechanism, dosage, adverse reactions, and special considerations please refer to the relevant literature. In principle, this field test does not claim against the principles of current and against overdosage compatibility principles of drug use.

c. Based on the principle of real reaction clinical events, summarizing the clinical results, if the vast majority of cases the use of a drug from a manufacturer, use the trade name of the drug, and the use of certain drugs are derived from multiple manufacturers use the common name of the drug.

d. The field test in a treatment plan or a drug sorting mainly reflects in the treatment of patients with effective or groups a treatment or drug use frequency, represents the developing trend of the current, the "sort" but with the deepening of the test and an increase in the number of cases and the influence factors, such as changing. So the existing order to provide a reference for the clinical diagnosis and treatment, also provide clinicians with a further understanding and practice of space.

e. Test results besides provide important information for clinical treatment, are also proved that the body symptoms of psychosomatic hypothesis to set up the chain of evidence classification are an important link.

Section 2   Classification of physical symptoms psychosomatic treatment results and interpretation

First, Psychosomatic medicine within the framework of the theory of classification of various body symptoms frequency and analysis treatment

a. The various types of body symptoms treatment results and statistics

About multi-center test research subjects in, exclusion criteria; the test research process; evaluation criteria such as information, refer to chapter 3. On into the group of patients on the basis of the clinical classification of somatic symptoms scale WCPA(R-1) after evaluation, reference, respectively, these recommendations or clinicians according to pathological physiology, pathology, psychological mechanism to the selected scheme for treatment, and after treatment of 4 weeks, 12 weeks follow-up, respectively, the aim was to evaluate the efficacy and the adverse effects of treatment, as well as other relevant information.The evaluation of curative effect in the clinical classification of somatic symptoms scale WCPA(R-1) points rate as the standard. According to the clinical standard, points rate is greater than or equal to 25% for effective, reduction rate is greater than or equal to 50% for signature. Results show that the use plan 4 weeks and 12 weeks when rating scale total score and each factor were significantly decreased ($P<0.001$) (Table 4-2-1).

**Table 4-2-1   Classification of somatic symptoms scale score results baseline,
4 weeks, 12 weeks**

items	baseline		4 weeks		12 weeks		F
	m	sd	m	sd	m	sd	P<0.001
Total Score	50.36	27.47	34.36	21.14	24.27	17.18	**
Inhibiting somatic symptom	51.41	27.99	35.57	21.35	24.16	16.22	**
Irritable somatic symptom	53.91	28.04	35.13	19.85	23.00	16.43	**
Biological somatic symptom	33.85	29.11	26.36	25.43	16.46	16.56	**
Imaginative somatic symptom	40.20	31.36	28.06	26.15	18.65	21.03	**
Cognitive somatic symptom	53.40	20.15	35.59	17.94	29.21	16.27	**

**note: treatmeat effect was significant that somatic symptoms significantly decreased at 1 month, 3 months after treatment.

From the results above, in the treatment of 12 weeks, for all kinds of somatic symptoms were significantly effective treatment.Statistics the recommendation at this time in all kinds of somatic symptoms in the frequency of treatment, and as an optimization scheme to preliminary promotion or as a symptom of perfecting the starting point of the clinical treatment plan is reasonable. The results of field test for true reflection treatment, treatment of drugs at the same time the use of multiple manufacturers still use the common name, while the single use of a drug manufacturer use the trade name of the manufacturer. In addition, because of considering the single type clinical symptoms of patients with less, usually based on a certain type symptom is given priority to, with or without symptoms of other types of group, so the recommended scheme is used more in combination, it will make different types of symptoms were alleviated; Inevitably, however, a combination of drugs will be added the frequency of the occurrence of adverse events, the clinical doctor comprehensive judging the pros and cons to make options. Reason to clinical practical need, when we in summary scheme respectively summarized every somatic types of single frequency sequence and joint scheme in frequency sorting.

b. The treatment of irritable somatic symptoms

Can be seen in the Table 4-2-1 and Table 4-2-1 in field test test in treatment of irritability somatic symptoms at 12 weeks single-agent scheme mainly SSRI drugs, sid (tandospirone) and SNRI drugs is given priority to, in composite scheme d force new pp (flupentixol and melitracen tablets) use frequency is highest, then is an SSRI or SNRI drugs as the core, and on this basis or a combination of benzodiazepines drugs (mainly long half-life of clonazepam) or combined with atypical antipsychotics (zyprexa or quetiapine flat highest frequency) or combined with another drug improves mood (with sid, shuganjieyu capsule, wuling capsule highest frequency). Field test results and we recommend ideas and solutions, and specific drugs in the recommended scheme of dose for clinical commonly used therapeutic doses. About the treatment and the drug use frequency of sorting, please see Table 4-2-2, Table 4-2-3, about the use of drugs by the daily dose see Table 4-2-4.

Table 4-2-2   Single drug in treatment of irritability body symptoms ranking

Frequency order	regimen
1	SSRIs drugs (specific drugs, in order: paroxetine hydrochloride, Lexapro (escitalopram citalopram), cipramil (citalopram), zoloft (sertraline hydrochloride)
2	SID (tandospirone)
3	SNRI class drugs followed by: cymbalta (duloxetine) or venlafaxine (venlafaxine)
4	Zyprexa (olanzapine)
5	Shugan Jieyu capsule

Table 4-2-3   **Treatment of patients with irritable symptoms combined ranking**

Frequency order	Regimen
1	Deanxit
2	SSRI drugs + clonazepam (SSRI drugs, in specific usage frequency order to at, Lexapro, paroxetine hydrochloride, zoloft and cipramil
3	SNRI class drugs + benzodiazepine drugs (SNRI drug use frequency were: venlafaxine, and cymbalta; specific benzodiazepine class drugs used were: clonazepam, and alprazolam)
4	SSRI drugs (use frequency were: lexapro, zoloft, paroxetine hydrochloride) + SID + atypical antipsychotic drugs (use frequency were: zyprexa, and quetiapine)
5	SSRI drugs (specific frequency of use is: lexapro, and fluoxetine "fluoxetine hydrochloride", and zoloft) + zyprexa
6	SSRI drugs (zoloft, paroxetine hydrochloride) + shugan jieyu capsules
7	SSRI drugs (zoloft, paroxetine hydrochloride) + wuling capsule

Table 4-2-4   **Treatment of irritable somatic symptoms drug regimen daily dose range**

Drug names	Daily dose range	Drug names	Daily dose range
Paroxetine hydroChloride	20-50mg	Deanxit	1-3 tablets
Lexapro	5-20mg	Venlafaxin	75-225mg
Fluoxetine	20-40mg	Zyprexa	2.5-10mg
Cymbalta	60-120mg	Quetiapine	50-100mg
Zoloft	100-150mg	Sid	15-45mg
Cipramil	20-40mg	Shuganjieyu capsules	720-1440mg
Clonazepam	1-3mg	Alprazolam	0.4-1.2mg
Wuling capsule	3-9 tablets		

c. The treatment of inhibiting the body symptoms

12 weeks of treatment plan of frequency sorting and drug dose range are shown in Table 4-2-5, Table4-2-6, Table 4-2-7. Displays the field test test the inhibitory somatic symptoms at 12 weeks single-agent scheme mainly SSRI drugs, sid and SNRI drugs use frequency is highest;The

composite scheme using frequency is in turn in her new, SSRI drugs and
SNRI combination of drugs as the core.In the treatment of inhibiting the
body symptoms, treatment of frequency and specific drugs and treatment
irritable somatic symptoms and specific drugs similar to analysis its reason mainly has the following several aspects: ①the previous related
studies show that high frequency solution used in all kinds of antidepressant and anti-anxiety drugs with the two aspects of the role, the role of
pathological anxiety, depression, two more accurate optimal treatment
produce subject to treat cases continue to accumulate; ②according to the
basic principle of psychology as well as to the thinking on the development process of abnormal emotion, anxiety should first be regarded as
basic emotion, is closely related to the normal physiological and psychological process.The occurrence of mood disorders to stress as a starting
point (including physiological stress and psychological stress), under the
action of "stress", individual produce anxiety. Put it on the anxiety, including psychological stress under the meaning of anxiety and somatic
stress level in the sense of anxiety.The former can appear such as described in the catalogs of mental illness of post-traumatic stress disorder,
generalized anxiety, panic disorder, social anxiety disorder, forced disorder, sleep disorder, etc, which can show the changes in blood pressure,
glucose metabolism, endocrine dysfunction, abnormal irritable digestive
symptoms, pain, and so on and so forth. In stress cannot be eliminated, or
on the basis of stress "secondary stress source" making individual continuous response to stress condition (such as individual tumors after tumors cause unemployment crisis, family relationship, family economic
situation in distress, and so on and so forth), or inappropriate response to
the crisis due to the individual character flaws such as cases, individual
anxiety state might as experience or as a body form exist for a long time.
And pathological anxiety long-standing result can appear two cases, one

is the anxiety of failure, characterized by lack of motivation, interest of
the individual which can depression, such as when individuals in a con-
stant state of stress, the activity of HPA axis, increased cortisol can lead to
some of the central nervous system structure such as the hippocampus
and the amygdala prefrontal cortex damage, leading to cognitive dysfunction, and pathological depression, and is reflected in the body, the inhibitory somatic symptoms. From the above according to the research on the
various aspects of inference that strong link between anxiety and depression, it is difficult to separate from, this is also because the irritable somatic symptoms and inhibitory somatic symptoms in treatment more similar to one of the reasons for treatment. In addition, according to the
above anxiety, depression, the analysis of the continuous process of the
development of the clinical diagnosis of patients with what is actual status
of judgment than for its labeled as a diagnostic term "label" has more
practical significance.Need to be more precise, of course, the premise of
optimization treatment has yet to be physical symptom classification continue to optimize the tool of the scale.

**Table 4-2-5   Therapeutic inhibition of somatic symptoms alone program
frequency**

Frequency sort	Therapeutic regimen
1	SSRI drugs (drug use frequency were: paroxetine hydrochloride, lexapro, cipramil, zoloft, fluoxetine
2	Sid
3	SNRI class drugs (drug use frequency were: cymbalta, and venlafaxine
4	Zyprexa
5	Shuganjieyu capsule
6	Wuling capsule

**Table 4-2-6   Therapeutic inhibition of somatic symptoms combined regimen
appears the frequency**

Frequency sort	Therapeutic regimen
1	Deanxit
2	SNRI class drugs + benzodiazepine drugs (SNRI drugs in specific frequency): venlafaxine, and cymbalta; specific drug of the benzodiazepine class drug use frequency were: alprazolam, and clonazepam)
3	SSRI drugs + benzodiazepines (SSRI drugs, in specific frequency order to lexapro, fluoxetine, and paroxetine hydrochloride, zoloft, cipramil
4	SNRI drugs + zyprexa, benzodiazepines drugs (including SNRI drugs specific drug concrete using frequency in the order: cymbalta, venlafaxine)
5	SSRI medications + zyprexa (including specific drug use frequency, in order: SSRI drugs to at, Lexapro, fluoxetine, zoloft)
6	SSRI medications + proprietary Chinese medicine (SSRI drugs specific drug use frequency, in order: zoloft, paroxetine hydrochloride; and proprietary chinese medicine: shuganjieyu capsule, wuling capsule)

Table 4-2-7   Inhibitory of somatic symptoms drug regimen of daily dose

Drug names	Daily dose range	Drug names	Daily dose range
Deanxit	1-3 tablets	Venlafaxine	75-225mg
Paroxetine hydrochloride	20-60mg	Sid	10-60mg
Zoloft	50-150mg	Zyprexa	2.5-15mg
Lexapro	10-20mg	Quetiapine	50-100mg
Cipramil	15-40mg	Clonazepam	1.5mg
Fluoxetine	20-40mg	Wuling capsule	3-9 tablets
Cymbalta	60-120mg	Shuganjieyu capsules	720-1440mg

d. For the treatment of cognitive somatic symptoms

12 weeks of treatment plan of frequency sorting and drug dose range are shown in Table 4-2-8, Table 4-2-9, Table 4-2-10. Field test tests for the treatment of cognitive somatic symptoms at 12 weeks single-agent ranking the highest frequency of alternative respectively the SSRI drugs, sid and cymbalta, followed by zyprexa. About cognitive symptoms, as as already described in the first section of this chapter, here refers to the

cognitive symptoms consist of two meanings, one is the negative interpretation of the body, the second refers to the physical symptoms consistent with illusion features. The two cases are closely associated with
individual cognitive dysfunction, so the goal of treatment should be given
priority should be to improve cognitive function, simultaneity, improve
the negative mood, in order to promote its symptoms disappear.Test frequency and basic conform to the selection of drug treatment concept.
Only in the sorting of drug use of antianxiety agents use frequency seems
to be higher than atypical antipsychotic drugs to improve cognitive function. The results indicate: ①conform to adjust mood is an important link
in improving cognitive function, on this view, please see the first chapter,
especially see the description of the cognitive level of anxiety; ②because
the drug use frequency is based on the statistics by 12 weeks after treatment to effective statistical case, it is necessary to reflect on the accuracy
of classification scale, namely in the later field test should further pay
attention to the difference between emotional and cognitive symptoms;
③understanding from the psychological perspective, cognitive process,
emotional process and will process are three interrelated cannot be sepa-
rated from the process of adjustment in the treatment of cognitive body
symptoms negative emotions of drugs and improve the cognition of drugs
used in combination in order to obtain better effect salience, just need to
be further accumulated treatment cases in order to more accurately reflect
the optimization of such symptoms.

Table 4-2-8   Treatment of cognitive symptoms alone program frequency

Frequency sort	Therapeutic regimen
1	SSRI medications (in specific drug sort order to at, zoloft)
2	Sid
3	Cymbalta
4	Zyprexa

Table 4-2-9   Treatment of cognitive symptoms combined regimen appears the frequency

Frequency sort	therapeutic regimen
1	Deanxit
2	SSRI medications, sid and atypical antipsychotics (SSRI drugs, in specific drug sort order zoloft, to at, paroxetine hydrochloride; atypical antipsychotics specific medication in the order: zyprexa, quetiapine)
3	Sid + benzodiazepines drugs (benzodiazepines drugs specific medication in the order: lorazepam, alprazolam)
4	SNRI drugs + sid + zyprexa (SNRI drugs specific medication order are: cymbalta, venlafaxine)
5	SSRI medications, atypical antipsychotics and benzodiazepines drugs (SSRI drugs, in specific drug sort order to at, paroxetine hydrochloride, zoloft; atypical antipsychotics, in the specific use of zyprexa, quetiapine; benzodiazepines drugs specific medication is: lorazepam, alprazolam)
6 Two schemes (the columns appear in actual test frequency is the same)	(1) SSRI drugs + zyprexa (SSRI drugs used in this scheme, in order: to at, paroxetine) (2) cymbalta + sid + benzodiazepines drugs (benzodiazepines drugs of specific drugs for: lorazepam, alprazolam)
7	Paroxetine + shuganjieyu capsule

Table 4-2-10   Cognitive somatoform symptoms daily dose

Drug names	Daily dose range	Drug names	Daily dose range
Zoloft	50-150mg	Zyprexa	1.25-10mg
Venlafaxine	75-150mg	Quetiapine	50mg
Cymbalta	60-120mg	Lorazepam	0.5mg qn
Cipramil	5-20mg	Alprazolam	0.2-0.8mg qn
Paroxetine hydrochloride	10-40mg	Shuganjieyu capsules	720-1440mg qd
Deanxit	0.5-3 tablets		
Lexapro	10-20mg		
Sid	10-30mg		

e. For the treatment of imaginary somatic symptoms

For imaginative treatment after 12 weeks of treatment plan of fre-

quency sorting and drug dose range are shown in Table 4-2-11, Table
4-2-12, Table 4-2-13. Statistical results show that the field test in treatment of imaginative somatic symptoms at 12 weeks, almost all effective
cases of single drug solution to SSRI drugs, SNRI drugs, wuling capsule,
shuganjieyu capsule improves mood of drugs;Also presents the trend basically combined regimen. As described in the first chapter, imaginative
somatic symptoms based on hints, self-suggestion, suggests that, in certain circumstances and in a certain emotional atmosphere, individual impact on from the outside to accept unconditionally. Individual is suggestive of the highest ages 5 to 7 years old, or generally speaking, should be
in the early stage of the youth, become a part of the individual personality
development is not mature. To mature adulthood as personality, implicit
and if in adulthood still maintained a nonage high suggestibility, this cre-
ates a personality based imaginative body symptoms.Treatment of imaginary somatic symptoms, therefore, the basic goal has two aspects, one is
to reduce the contrast, the second is to improve the cognitive function.
Anti-anxiety drugs can reduce a person's alertness, and thus can reduce
its suggestibility, while atypical antipsychotic drugs can improve cognitive function, which is in the two types of drug use in the scene test frequency is high, and multiple test unit medicine direction are consistent.
As to whether or not is given priority to with anti-anxiety drugs and the
treatment with atypical antipsychotics was quite the best treatment to be
physical symptoms continue to accumulate cases. It is worth to mention
again at the same time, according to the imaginary somatic symptoms
pathological psychological foundation, the treatment of this kind of
symptom besides medication, psychological counseling should be treated
is an important link. For this problem is also subject to treat cases continue to accumulate.

Table 4-2-11   Treatment of imagined somatic symptoms alone program frequency

Drug use frequency sorting	Regimen
1	SSRI medications (specific drug use frequency, in order: Lexapro, zoloft, ciprami
2	SNRI drugs (specific drugs in use the sort order: cymbalta, venlafaxine)
3	Wuling capsule
4	Shuganjieyu capsules

Table 4-2-12   Treatment of imagined physical symptoms combined regimen appears the frequency

Drug use frequency sorting	Regimen
1	Deanxit
2	SSRI drugs + SID + atypical antipsychotic drugs (SSRI drugs drug use frequency were: zoloft, paroxetine hydrochloride, lexapro; Atypical antipsychotics in specific frequency: olanzapine, and quetiapine, and aripiprazole tablets)
3	SID + benzodiazepine drugs (drugs in turn, to lorazepam, alprazolam)
4 (The same frequency of the two options set out in the column the same)	SNRI class drugs + benzodiazepine drugs (SNRI class drugs drugs are: cymbalta, and venlafaxine; benzodiazepines drugs to specific drugs, in order: lorazepam, alprazolam)
	+ SSRI drug benzodiazepine drugs (SSRI drugs drug use were: paroxetine hydrochloride, cipramil, lexapro; benzodiazepine drugs drug use were: lorazepam, alprazolam)
5	SNRI class drugs atypical antipsychotic drugs + benzodiazepine drugs (SNRI class drugs drug use in this scenario is mainly cymbalta atypical antipsychotic drugs followed by quetiapine, olanzapine; benzodiazepine drugs followed by lorazepam, and alprazolam)

Table 4-2-13   Treatment of somatic symptoms using drugs daily dose

Drug names	Daily dose range	Drug names	Daily dose range
zoloft	100-150mg	Quetiapine	12.5-50mg
Paroxetine hydrochloride	30-50mg	Zyprexa	2.5-10mg
Cymbalta	30-60mg	Aripiprazole tablets	5-10mg
Lexapro	5-20mg	Deanxit	1-2 tablets
Cipramil	20-40mg	Shuganjieyu capsules	720-1440mg
Venlafaxine	75-225mg	Wuling capsule	3-9 tablets
Zyprexa	2.5-7.5mg qn	Lorazepam	0.5-1.5mg
Sid	20-60mg qd	Alprazolam	0.2-0.8mg qn

f. For biological treatment of somatic symptoms

12 weeks of treatment plan of frequency sorting and drug dose range are shown in Table 4-2-14, Table 4-2-15, Table 4-2-16. Results show that the field test the biological body symptoms at 12 weeks single-agent scheme almost all with SSRI drugs, SNRI drugs, Diane force new, benzodiazepines drugs, and shuganjieyu capsule, wu ling capsule have anti-anxiety effect of drugs. Described by this and the first chapter of the meaning of "biological physical symptoms", admitted the pathological damage in the role of this kind of symptom, and emphasize individual cognition, emotion, personality and real life situation to produce symptoms or impact on the severity of symptoms. Therefore, the biological treatment of somatoform symptoms should include two parts, one is the treatment of pathological damage, but the mental state of patient evaluation and give the corresponding treatment. From a biological standpoint, negative experience of the generation mechanism and uplink system is activated and central nervous system is directly related to the derepression downlink systems, and the uplink system is activated and downlink system is to take off the curb and closely related to psychological factors, especially closely associated with emotional factors. Such as in the in-

tense atmosphere of the war, because war individual under high stress
state of passion, produced by the injury, is even more severe damage can
be is the best example.In this test, therefore, the use of anti-anxiety drugs
reduce a person's alert level, make produced by pathological damage of
sexual experience to reduce or even eliminate the salience. Used for such
symptoms, then, at the same time also have the function of antidepressant
drugs, reduce the body symptoms are associated with antidepressant effects?The judgment is unlikely, because depression pathological mental
process is led to the decrease of the individual alertness, allowing it to
from their own or outside, the sensitivity of the drop in the condition of
the natural negative experience degree will decline, pathological state of
extreme depression is "depressive stupor" , the individual to external
stimulation or serious damage to the basic no physiological or psychological response. According to the result of field test, at least for the moment can be concluded that the treatment of biological body symptoms of
psychosomatic development is the basic principle of treatment of pathological injury on the basis of the combined use of certain types of anti-anxiety drugs. As for the treatment of biological body symptom more
accurate use of anti-anxiety drugs, whether for some patients also need to
focus on improving cognition and whether the use of sedative hypnotic
drugs in patients with some or whether can also support the use of counseling problems to be further accumulation treatment cases. In addition,
as a true reflection of clinical events, clinical treatment of biological body
symptoms found in testing SSRI drugs + deanxit force new treatment,
statistics found that the scheme of using high frequency, and effective.
But her new tricyclic antidepressants ingredients and typical antipsychotic drug ingredients, is a joint preparation, already have anti-anxiety effect,
at the same time, it has to improve cognitive function, and combined use of
SSRI drugs does not seem to be necessary, at the same time tricyclic drug

combination SSRI drugs have an increased risk of adverse reactions.In view of the foregoing reasons, should not be the treatment plan for future clinical practice biological body symptoms or other kind of somatic symptoms treatment recommendations, so it is not in the order listed in the table.

Table 4-2-14   Treatment of bio-physical symptoms as monotherapy program frequency

The frequency sequence	Regimen
1	SSRI medications (specific frequency in the order: zoloft, Lexapro, paroxetine hydrochloride, cipramil
2	SNRI drugs (specific frequency in the order: cymbalta, venlafaxine
3	Shuganjieyu capsules
4	Wuling capsule

Table 4-2-15   Treatment of biological body symptoms frequency combination scheme

The frequency sequence	Regimen
1	Deanxit
2	Cymbalta + zyprexa + clonazepam
3	Zoloft + benzodiazepines drugs (specific frequency in the order: clonazepam, alprazolam, lorazepam)

Table 4-2-16   Daily dose for the treatment of biological body symptoms specific drug

Drug names	Daily dose range	Drug names	Daily dose range
Zoloft	50-150mg	Deanxit	1-2 tablets
Venlafaxine	75-225mg	Sid	10mg
Cipramil	20-60mg	Alprazolam	0.2-0.4mg
Paroxetine hydrochloride	20-60mg	Lorazepam	0.5-1mg
Lexapro	15-20mg	Clonazepam	1-2mg
Shuganjieyu capsules	1440mg	Wuling capsule	3-9 tablets

Second, the recommended scheme of adverse reactions

After treatment of 4 weeks, reports of adverse reaction followed by dry mouth, constipation, drowsiness, muscle stiffness, adverse reactions after 12 weeks sorting for constipation, dry mouth, weight gain, headaches. Not found in the clinical observation of the adverse reactions described above will affect individual social function or endanger the health conditions, so in general, the recommended scheme was proved to be safe. In addition, what kind of treatment to the clinician to choose comprehensive evaluation and treatment of patients with specific targets.

Third, the test results should be noted on the spot questions

a. According to the therapeutic effect and the frequency in the case of relatively large treatment, more than the recommended scheme can be used as an optimization scheme used in clinical treatment. But all the recommendations for the team to participate in the custom consensus and adoption, there may be a known limitations as well as the limitations of clinical experience, so the "optimization" treatment only represent the results of 2014-2016, and in a broader range of clinical practice and further optimization of treatment is necessary.

b. In the emotional body symptoms and cognitive body symptoms of all the schemes, appear with valproate zyban, Valproic acid magnesium zyban, lamotrigine single-agent scheme and its combination with other drugs, and effective treatment results. Because this kind of drugs is not within the recommended scheme, at the same time, the frequency is low, in this not in the order listed in the table. But this is a notable trend, because the drugs belong to mood stabilizers, according to the research data show that in recent years, the drugs have the function of the stable biological rhythms, stable state of mind is just one aspect of their function. Therefore future work should continue to pay attention to accumulate the case of a mood stabilizer treatment, to explore whether there is "rhythmic body symptoms".

(Xueli Sun; Fanmin Zeng)

Section 3   The case of all kinds of physical symptom treatment

Case 1: the pain as the main symptoms of cognitive somatic case

Liu was a 35-year-old married man with main complaint of prickling on left forearm for 2 years. He got his upper left forearm slightly scratched with swelling, pain, and no bleeding in a traffic accident 2 years ago. Swelling subsidised and pain relieved after alcohol disinfection treatment by himself. Half a month later, he felt prickling on his left forearm whenever touched clothes which had later progressed into all kinds of objects. It felt like that there were numerous needles lined up pricking his skin with continuous slight pain, and could relive after removing the objects. Although the symptoms were slight and the pain was tolerable with no impact on sleep, his mood was terribly affected with influence on work and daily life so he had visited several hospitals. Physical examination results showed no malformation, mass, swelling or hot pain on the left arm and myodynamia, muscle tension and limb activity were normal. Examination results of X-ray, MRI for arms and neck, and electrophysiological showed no significant abnormal. The preliminary diagnosis was "pain to be determined". After applied with a topical analgetic Fastum Gel, then oral agents of aspirin and ibuprofen with combination of light therapy and thermotherapy, pain partly relieved while prickling remained. Then we prescribed olanzapine 10 mg/day in consideration of the relationship between the symptoms and cognition. Prickling relieved and pain disappeared after 2 weeks' treatment. The patient totally recovered 3 weeks later.

Experience: when analysing the symptoms, it tended to attribute the chronic pain to the injury because acanthesthesia occurred after the accident. In view of no positive findings in physical and laboratory examinations and no obvious relief after given analgetics, we excluded inflammatory pain and neuropathological pain. When considered the characteristics of these symptoms listed below: i) acanthesthesia in line with hallucination occurring in the absence of a certain acupuncture, ii) no change of the complaint and location, iii) clearly described symptoms, iv) no definite pathophysiological factors, we believed that cognition might be the cause of the patient's discomfort and treatment should aim at cognition improvement. When considered the outcomes, olanzapine, an antipsychotic could improve cognition, exerted a significant improving effect on the patient's somatic symptoms rather than analgetics and physicotherapeutics indicating that the symptoms were probably cognitive somatic.

Case 2: characterized by hallucinations cognitive body symptoms

Wang was a 40-year-old married man with main complaint of a feeling trampling on cobblestones in right foot for 4 years. The patient, with no obvious cause, had a feeling that his right foot was trampling on sharp cobblestones when walking even on flat ground accompanied with pain 4 years ago. The symptom could disappear when aparted from the ground. Althought the pain was tolerable, the symptoms caused claudication and terribly impacted his mood, with influence on work and daily life. He had visited several hospitals. Physical examination results showed no malformation, mass, swelling or hot pain on lower limbs with normal myodynamia, muscle tension and limb activity. Examination results of X-ray, MRI for lower limbs, and electrophysiological showed no significant abnormal. The preliminary diagnosis was "paresthesia on right lower limb to be determined". There was no significant effect of Fastum

Gel and aspirin with combination of light therapy and thermotherapy. In view of the pain, irritative symptom was considered and buspirone 30 mg/day were prescribed for anxiety. However, the symptoms did not improve. After reanalysis, we believed that the feeling of trampling on cobblestones was in line with hallucination, and olanzapine 15mg/day was prescribed. After 2 weeks' treatment, the feeling had changed from trampling on cobblestones to sand and finally disappeared at week 5.

Experience: when analyse the symptoms, the main complaint was patient's subjective feeling of trampling on cobblestones accompanied with pain. However in clinical practice, clinicians tended to focus on the pain rather than patien's subjective feeling. In view of no positive findings in physical and laboratory examinations and no obvious relief after given analgetics, inflammatory pain and neuropathological pain were denied. When considered the characteristics of the symtom listed below: i) a feeling of trampling on cobblestones in line with hallucination even in the absence of a real cobblestone; ii) no change of the complaint and location; iii) clearly described symptoms; iv) no definite pathophysiological factors, we believed cognition might be the cause for the somatic symtom and treatment should aim at changing patient's cognition. When considered the outcomes, a significant improving effect of agents for hallucination was observed indicating that the symptom was probably cognitive somatic.

Case 3: cognitive symptoms characterized by abnormal sensation case

Li was a 39-year-old unemployed female with main complaint of strips churning in her head for 6 months and depression and anxiety for 3 months. Six months ago, with no obvious cause, the patient felt dizzy and fullness in her head with a feeling that some strips churning in it, accompanied with chest tightness, shortness of breath, palpitation, intermittent restless, nausea and poor sleep quality of difficulty falling asleep and waking during sleep. The strips churning feeling was clear, vivid and relatively fixed, aggravated when changing body position. She had visited the neurology department in a local hospital and the physical examination on nervous system and examination results of MRI indicating "no organic disease". The patient was then treated with neurotrophins and vasodilators, and no improvement was observed. She disbelieved the statement of "no organic disease" and depression, anxiety, interest decreasing and worries about somatic symptoms appeared 3 months ago. The patient visited the psychiatric outpatient of West China Hospital and was diagnosed with "somatoform disorder". The assessment results of WCPA Somatic Symptom Classification Scale for the first time were 1.50 for irritable somatic symptoms factor, 1.50 for inhibitory somatic symptoms factor, 1.40 for imaginative somatic symptoms factor, 0.80 for biological somatic symptoms factor, and 1.40 for cognitive somatic symptoms factor. All the laboratory examination results of thyroid function, cortisol, corticotropin, sex hormone and oral glucose tolerance test (OGTT) were within normal ranges. Cymbalta 60-90mg/day, olanzapine 2.5-5mg/day and clonazepam 1.0-3.0mg/day were prescribed for emotional somatic symptoms. One month later, despite significant relief of depression and anxiety, disappearance of shortness breath and palpitation and improvement on sleep quality, the patient still felt strips churning in her head with noise of snap and a screech of metal. Second assessment results of WCPA Somatic Symptom Classification Scale were 0.36 for irritable somatic symptoms factor, 0.67 for inhibitory somatic symptoms factor, 0.21 for imaginative somatic symptoms factor, 0 for biological somatic symptoms factor, and 1.20 for cognitive somatic symptoms factor. Olanzapine was increased to 10mg/day due to a significant high score of cognitive somatic symptoms factor. Two months later, the patient reported totally relieved on depres-

sion and anxiety and the churning feeling decreased by 70%. The patient
accepted treatment for less than 3 months so far.

Experience: the patient initially presented somatic symptoms of
strips churning in head with a screech of metal and visited our clinic due
to no improvement for a long time and accompanied terrible depression
and anxiety. Since the emotional factor was significant in Somatic Symptom Classification Scale, it tended to misdiagnosed as a kind of mood
disorder and prescribed antidepressant alone. In view of the longer experience of somatic symptoms and accompanied mood symptoms, the patient was given SNRIs for somatic symptoms, depression and anxiety, and
lower-dose atypical antipsychotics for cognition, anxiety and sleep problems. Mood symptoms significantly improved, while cognitive somatic
symptoms which were described as vivid and relatively fixed turned to be
the main problem. After increasing the dose of olanzapine, the patient's
cognition significantly improved. In conclusion, patients' symptoms are
often complicated and there can be a main symptom accompanied by
others, therefore treatment should not be limited. In order to achieve a
better clinical effect, a more appropriate therapy strategy of drugs and
dosage should be taken into account according to the objective results of
WCPA Somatic Symptom Classification Scale.

Case 4: irritable + cognitive body symptoms

Ma was a 31-year-old male worker with complaints of intermittent
limb numbness for 7 years and a feeling of muscle twitching for 5 years.
Seven years ago, the patient gradually felt numbness on his hands and
feet which continued for several minutes each time and occurred twice to
three times a month. Five years ago, the symptoms grew worse that he
failed to hold objects when numbness attacked and he began to feel muscle twitching on his arms, back and lower limbs which occurred several
times a month at the beginning and became more frequently when weath-

er changed. Half a year ago, the symptoms became further worse with pain when numbness attacked and muscle twitching occurred three to four times a day. During that period, the patient experienced increased dreaming, light sleep of frequently awoken by the numbness, energy loss in the day-time, palpitation and restless. He did so care about these symptoms that he felt he had suffered serious disease, and frequently visited departments of neurology, neurosurgery and Traditional Chinese Medicine (TCM). No abnormal result was found in examinations of muscle electrophysiology, X-ray of thoracic vertebra and lumbar vertebra, MRI of cervical vertebra and thoracic vertebra, and CT scan of the head. No improvement was observed after inpatient treatment for several times. Later, the patient visited us and was diagnosed with anxiety disorder. The first assessment results of WCPA Somatic Symptom Classification Scale were 1.08 for inhibitory somatic symptoms, 1.71 for irritable somatic symptoms factor, 0.20 for biological somatic symptoms factor, 1.80 for imaginative somatic symptoms factor, and 1.29 for cognitive somatic symptoms factor. The results of the Big Five Personality Inventory were 3.9 for neuroticism, 3.4 for extraversion, 2.8 for openness to experience, 3.0 for agreeableness and 3.2 for conscientiousness. The patient was then treated with cymbalta 60-120mg/day, seroquel 100-200mg/day, clonazepam 0-3mg/day combined with psychotherapy.

After 4 weeks' treatment, numbness significantly improved and there was still a feeling of muscle twitching without impact on daily life. The results of WCPA Somatic Symptom Classification Scale were 0.08 for inhibitory somatic symptoms, 0.70 for irritable somatic symptoms factor, 0 for biological somatic symptoms factor, 0.80 for imaginative somatic symptoms factor, and 0.21 for cognitive somatic symptoms factor. Three month later, the patient reported stable mood and numbness totally disappeared with somewhat muscle twitching feeling and believed that he was a normal person. The results of WCPA Somatic Symptom Classification Scale were 0 for inhibitory somatic symptoms, 0.14 for irritable somatic symptoms factor, 0 for biological somatic symptoms factor, 0.20 for imaginative somatic symptoms factor, and 0.14 for cognitive somatic symptoms factor.

Laboratory examination of endocrine system.

Results for baseline: TSH 0.857mU/L, T_3 1.52nmol/L, T_4 101.5nmol/L, FT_3 4.32pmol/L, FT_4 18.63pmol/L, ACTH 44.64pmol/L and cortisol 632.8nmol/L. Resutls after 3 months' treatment: TSH 2.44mU/L, T_3 1.89 nmol/L, T_4 119.8nmol/L, FT_3 5.52 pmol/L, FT_4 17.62 pmol/L, ACTH 19.30pmol/L and cortisol 503.6nmol/L.

Experience: when analyse the symptoms, they were identified as following characteristics, i) multi-position and diversiform, ii) unexplained and incurable by other special departments except psychiatry, iii) social function being affected, and iv) with biological symptoms of poor sleep, palpitation and restless. Patients with above characteristics should be considered the possibility of anxiety disorder. The symptoms of numbness, pain, muscle twitching and palpitation could be explained by somatic anxious symptoms.

In addition, the patient did have anxious emotion during that period. He felt like suffering serious disease and repeatedly visited hospital, and the symptoms worsened while weather changed and were more and more diversiform, which could be explained as imaginative somatic symptoms. After screened as imaginative and irritable symptoms by WCPA Somatic Symptom Classification Scale, the patient was given recommened regimens of anxiolytics plus atypical antipsychotics combined with psychotherapy which showed significant effective. When retesting WCPA Somatic Symptom Classification Scale 3 months later, both imaginative and irritable symptoms significantly decreased and the patient felt good.

Therefore, we suggested a comprehensive analysis and symptom assessment for patients with somatic symptoms in order to make a better therapeutic choice. In addition, for the body symptom classification scale the interpretation of the results, in addition to pay attention to the main symptoms are arranged in the first, also should pay attention to prompt the remaining few symptoms scores, especially should pay attention to score the second symptoms.First, the scores of cases irritable somatic symptoms and cognitive somatic symptoms scored the second, so the SNRI drugs + of atypical antipsychotics treatment should is the key to obtain curative effect.

Case 5: the pain as the main characteristics of irritable somatic symptoms

Yang was a 55-years-old woman, was admitted to department of rheumatology and immunology with a history of systemic pain for 3 years, deteriorating with ants crawling sensation for 2 months. Three years ago, the patient began to fell limb muscle pain, limited mobility and numbness in the hands and feet. Antinuclear antibody was ++1:1000 while complement was C3 0.6970 g/L during her hospitalization. Bone density examination showed osteoporosis. Lip gland biopsy showed mild chronic inflammation of underlip mucosa with squamous cell hyperplasia, only a small lobulated salivary gland tissue was seen, part of the salivary gland acinar cells decreased or disappeared with fibrous tissue hyperplasia. The diagnoses were Sjogren's syndrome and Osteoporosis. The symptoms greatly improved after prednisone and anetholtrithione were given. One year ago, with no obvious cause, the patient felt pain in right chest and back which were not related to breathing with long term insomnia. She was diagnosed as "Sjogren's syndrome, fibromyalgia syndrome, white matter demyelination, pulmonary infection and osteoporosis" and prednisone, methylprednisolone, cyclophosphamide, pregabalin, cefmetazole sodium and supportive treatment including calcium supplement, gastric mucosa protecting and improving microcirculation were applied. The patient improved and discharged soon. Two months ago, the patient was admitted to hospital again with the similar symptoms reappeared, however she did not show any improvement after treatment as Sjogren's syndrome. The results of WCPA Somatic Symptom Classification Scale were 2.93 for irritable somatic symptoms, 2.92 for inhibitory somatic symptoms factor, 2.4 for imaginative somatic symptoms factor, 1.60 for biological somatic symptoms factor, and 1.30 for cognitive somatic symptoms factor. All the laboratory examination results of thyroid function, cortisol, corticotropin, sex hormone and oral glucose tolerance test (OGTT) were within normal ranges. Cymbalta, tiapride, olanzapine, clonazepam were given based on the somatic symptoms classification, and symptoms improved significantly after 1 month treatment. Second assessment results of WCPA Somatic Symptom Classification Scale were 1.85 for irritable somatic symptoms, 2.00 for inhibitory somatic symptoms factor, 1.60 for imaginative somatic symptoms factor, 0.80 for biological somatic symptoms factor, and 0.93 for cognitive somatic symptoms factor. The pain symptom almost disappeared after 2 months treatment, and only interest was not fully recovered. The patient accepted treatment for less than 3 months so far.

Experience: although this patient was diagnosed as Sjogren's syndrome, her systemic pain could not be explained by the diagnosis. Treatment should not be limited to biological treatment. Based on the theory of psychosomatic medicine, her systemic pain and ants crawling sensation belonged to irritable somatic symptoms. According to the results of Somatic Symptom Classification Scale, irritable and inhibitory somatic symptoms factors were top two effected factors. After treating with cymbalta, tiapride, olanzapine and clonazepam for emotional somatic symptoms, the patient got improvement.

Case 6: characterized by such hallucinations of imaginary body case

Huang was a 55-year-old dancer, started to feel all his joints were loose and dislocated 4 years ago. When he moved, he felt his spine elongated, shoulder joint displaced, local muscle stretched, weakness and blood stream running inside his vessels sometimes. These feelings prevented him from moving. He visited neurosurgery clinic and went through the spine X-ray and MRI scan for his neck and shoulders, all results were negative. He started to worry about these symptoms all day long, which in turn caused him even more problems such as palpitations, sweating and palm fever. Three years ago, he visited psychiatric clinic in mental health center of West China Hospital and was diagnosed as "schizophrenia". He got no respond to treatment of risperidone 5mg/day and olanzapine 2.5mg/night. He had to lie in bed all day because moving his body made him feel worse. Moreover, he felt his muscles were twisting from his feet moving up to head, and his bones and muscles were loose. He was then hospitalized in psychosomatic department of our hospital and was diagnosed as "somatoform disorder". The frist assessment results of WCPA Somatic Symptom Classification Scale were 0.75 for inhibitory somatic symptoms, 1.21 for irritable somatic symptoms factor, 0.20 for biological somatic symptoms factor, 2.60 for imaginative somatic symptoms factor, and 1.00 for cognitive somatic symptoms factor. The results of the Big Five Personality Inventory were 1.83 for neuroticism, 4.25 for extraversion, 3.17 for openness to experience, 3.67 for agreeableness and 4.17 for conscientiousness. He was treated with cymbalta 60-120mg/day, quetiapine 200-800mg/day and tandospirone 15mg-30mg/day, combined with psychotherapy and suggestive therapy. Four weeks later, the patient reported a "slight" change that his felt less worry and his twisted muscles did not limit his movement anymore. Second assessment results of WCPA Somatic Symptom Classification Scale were 0 for inhibitory somatic symptoms, 0.07 for irritable somatic symptoms factor, 0 for biological somatic symptoms factor, 1.67 for imaginative somatic symptoms factor, and 0.29 for cognitive somatic symptoms factor. After 3 months treatment, the patient reported his mood was stable, physical discomfort was relieved, with only a few muscles in the back still twisted occasionally which did not affect his activity. The last assessment results of WCPA Somatic Symptom Classification Scale were 0 for inhibitory somatic symptoms, 0.07 for irritable somatic symptoms factor, 0 for biological somatic symptoms factor, 1.3 for imaginative somatic symptoms factor, and 0.14 for cognitive somatic symptoms factor.

Laboratory examination of endocrine system.

Results for baseline: TSH 3.997mU/L, T_3 1.207nmol/L, T_4 90.606 nmol/L, FT_3 5.241pmol/L, FT_4 14.218 pmol/L, ACTH 40.28 pmol/L, cortisol 566.2 nmol/L. Results after 3 months' treatment: TSH 4.259 mU/L, T_3 0.987 nmol/L, T_4 54.068 nmol/L, FT_3 5.344 pmol/L, FT_4 8.509 pmol/L, ACTH 19.20 pmol/L, CORT 439.2 nmol/L.

Experience: this patient's symptoms were muscles twisting and bones loose. We firstly diagnosed him as schizophrenia because we took the symptoms as visceral hallucination. The patient didn't respond to a standard schizophrenic treatment so we reanalyzed his symptoms. Firstly, his symptoms were varied both in location and in property. Secondly, taking his personality into account, he was a dancer, and was emotional and dramatic. Thirdly, WCPA Somatic Symptom Classification Scale showed he had imaginative somatic symptoms. Imaginative somatic symptoms due to suggest and self-talk, which is associated with cognitive dysfunction, also associated with negative emotions, so, Base on these considerations, we used the recommended treatment rigimen antianxietics plus atypical antipsychotics, combined with psychotherapy and suggestive therapy, which had much better effect than using antipsychotics alone. After 3 months treatment, the imaginative somatic symptoms score decreased obviously. In addition, while he felt his muscles twisting, he also experienced anxiety. This was confirmed in the first assessment results and the reason we gave him antianxietics. After 3 month treatment, the irritation somatic symptoms score had decreased too.

In brief, the most important thing was to grasp its essence comprehensively when we analyzed patients' somatic symptoms. Meanwhile, proper tools, like WCPA Somatic Symptom Classification Scale and personality scales, could help us filter the core symptoms and evaluate efficacy and outcome quantitatively.

Case 7: inhibitory somatic symptoms of rhythm characteristics

Liu is a 27-year-old female with main complaint of repeated loss of consciousness with twitching limbs for more than 10 years and depression with waning interest for 5 years. Ten years ago, she was diagnosed as epilepsy and the characteristic of the clinical seisures was comprehensive tetanic convulsion with the frequency of 2-3 times/month. She had used carbamazepine, Depakine, levetiracetam and other kind of drugs for treatment, the therapy effect was unsatisfied though the dosage was adjusted repeatedly during the ten years. Five years ago, the patient began to feel depressed emotion with loss of interest in things and had insomnia as early awakening. She also felt poor spirit and malaise during daytime, suicidal ideation may appear when it was severe. Besides, she was diagnosed as Polycystic ovary syndrome (PCOS) because of the long-term irregular menstrual cycle. Those symptoms had seriously affected the patient's social function, as a result, she was break at home for nearly ten years. During her hospitalization in the department of neurology, both the medical and neurological examination showed no abnormalities. Auxiliary examination: long-range video electroencephalogram (VEEG) reminded severe abnormalities; thyroid function showed an increase in TSH and the Hamilton Depression Scale (HAMD) score was 22. The first assessment results of WCPA Somatic Symptom Classification Scale were 2.4 for inhibitory somatic symptoms factor, 1.9 for irritable somatic symptoms factor, 1.6 for biological somatic symptoms factor, 0.9 for imaginative somatic symptoms factor and 1.3 for cognitive somatic symptoms factor.As the main kind was biological somatic symptoms factor, we gave depakine 500mg bid, kaplan 500mg bid, cipramil 20mg qd and other drugs for treatment.

After 4 weeks' treatment, the patient felt much better emotion and the seizure frequency was reduced from three times last month to only once the next month. The results of reexamination of sex hormones, thyroid function, blood lipids, OGTT and gynecological ultrasound were all normal; the HAMD score decreased from 22 to 14 with the total score of somatic symptoms decreased from 8.1 to 2.3. Overall evaluation of its curative effect should be seen as "*". At present in the continue treatment.

Treatment experience: basic treatment for the patient to use: antiepileptic drugs (mood stabilizer) + SSRI medications, and treatment effect is depression, seizures, and polycystic ovary syndrome in biological indicator, depression, or as an experience negative feelings of somatic symptoms were improved significantly. It has to imagine that should exist the possibility of some kind of inner link between the three.Review foreign related research literature suggests that pathological depressive mood belongs to the emotional rhythm abnormalities, epilepsy electric circadian rhythm abnormalities, central nervous system and polycystic ovary syndrome is the result of HPA axis rhythm abnormalities, as the main mood stabilizers of antiepileptic drug plays an important role in stability and adjust the biological rhythm, three kinds of situations and should alleviate the key lies in the core function of the biological rhythm adjustment while SSRI drugs in the treatment of patients with this case should also played an important supporting role. This case should be associated with the problem in the clinical diagnosis and treatment, should pay attention to dysrhythmia problem, at the same time, for classification of somatic symptoms, should pay attention to in future clinical practice dedicated to exist the possibility of "rhythmic body symptoms".

Case 8: irritable somatic symptoms characteristic of rhythm

Xiao was a 15-years-old Junior Three student with main complaint of recurrent abdominalgia for 5 months. Five months ago, the first day of participated in military training, the patient began to vomiting stomach contents, about 3-4 times a day, no other associated symptoms. After 7 days symptomatic treatment of "acute gastroenteritis" at a local hospital, vomiting improved, while abdominal pain began. He felt upper and left abdominal persistent angina, no radiation pain and no accompanying symptoms, intensified after eating. The results of abdominal X-ray indicating "ileus" ? After symptomatic treatment, vomiting disappeared and the pain persisted. He was then hospitalized in gastroenterology department of West China Hospital. Examination results of abdominal ultrasound and enhanced CT, small bowel barium meal showed on significant abnormal. Gastroscopy showed that there was a flake erythema at the greater curvature of the middle of gastric body. Colonoscopy showed the terminal ileitis and proctitis. Terminal ileum pathological examination reported that moderate chronic inflammation of mucous, lymphoid follicular formation. After a general discussion, gastroenterology department considered "Purpura enteropathy", and used methylprednisolone pulse therapy. He was discharged from hospital after abdominal pain relieved. One week later, the pain was back. He reported upper and left abdominal persistent and fixed angina. The pain was paroxysmal aggravation, as well as full abdominal tenderness. He hospitalized in gastroenterology department again. There was no significant effect of pulse therapy. Laboratory examination: The "three great regular tests" showed leukocyte count 3.32 $\times 10^9$/L↓, others was normal. Liver and renal functions, stool routine test, urine routine test, ACTH, thyroid function, thyroid antibodies, thyroid ultrasound, ECG were normal. PTC(8-10) 11.26 nmol/L↓. The assessment results of WCPA Somatic Symptom Classification Scale for the first time were 0.33 for inhibitory somatic symptoms factor, 0.93 for irritable somatic symptoms factor, 0 for biological somatic symptoms factor, 0.36 for imaginative somatic symptoms factor, 0.7 for cognitive somatic symptoms factor, the total score 29. He was treated with cymbalta 30mg tid, tiapride 100mg tid, olanzapine 5mg qn, depakine 500mg qd, clonazepam 1mg tid. One week later, the patient reported abdominal pain disappeared, anxiety and sleep symptoms were improved significantly. Four weeks later, abdominal pain didn't recurrence. Second assessment results of WCPA Somatic Symptom Classification Scale were 0.08 for inhibitory somatic symptoms factor, 0.12 for irritable somatic symptoms factor, 0 for biological somatic symptoms factor, 0.07 for imaginative somatic symptoms factor, 0.3 for cognitive somatic symptoms factor, the total score 8. After 3 months treatment, the patient reported vomiting didn't recurrence. The last assessment results of WCPA Somatic Symptom Classification Scale were 0 for inhibitory somatic symptoms factor, 0.07 for irritable somatic symptoms factor, 0 for biological somatic symptoms factor, 0 for imaginative somatic symptoms factor, 0.1 for cognitive somatic symptoms factor, the total score 2. Reviewed TSH 1.930 mU/L, T_3 1.4 nmol/L, T_4 99.47 nmol/L, FT_3 3.60 pmol/L, FT_4 20.20 pmol/L, ACTH 76.14 pmol/L, PTC 397.60 nmol/L。

Experience: summarize the key to success lies in the diagnosis and treatment of patients with somatic symptoms of patients with interpreting the concept of lack of medical and setbacks of the key is early diagnosis and treatment may exist only to repeatedly find the patient's pathology and ignored the interpretation of symptoms. Summarize the key to success lies in the diagnosis and treatment of patients with somatic symptoms of patients with interpreting the concept of lack of medical and setbacks of the key is early diagnosis and treatment may exist only to repeatedly find the patient's pathology and ignored the interpretation of symptoms.The classification of somatic symptoms scale evaluation results suggest the nature of the symptoms of the patient is irritable somatic symptoms, but only this is not enough, again combing the history data found that patients with the irritable somatic symptoms with rhythmic features, thus making the treatment plan for mood stabilizer + SNRI drugs, atypical antipsychotics, treat mood stabilizer's goal is to adjust the rhythm, SNRI drugs to fight anxiety and depression, with atypical antipsychotic drugs to improve cognitive function, and obtain good effect.With seven cases by the same token, the process of diagnosis and treatment of this case indicate whether there is a separate rhythmic body symptoms, is worth in clinical practice for the future to further accumulate treatment cases.

Case 9: imaginative examples of physical symptoms associated with irritable symptoms

Yang was a 56-year-old retired woman, with no obvious cause, started to have trouble to fall asleep 2 years ago. She ignored that as it is light. Then she gradually felt bloating, bellyache. The pain's location was changed, and radiated to the back, accompanied with stomach fever, acid regurgitation, dizziness, palpitation, sweating, and limb numbness, and reduced when she closed her eyes. She urinated normally, while dyschesia, constipine, and had to take laxatives. After frequently visited local hospital, no abnormal pathological changes were found. She went to many hospitals as the symptoms terribly impacted her mood and influence on daily life. 4 months ago, other hospital considered "intestine adhesion" and given "enterolysis", no improvement was observed. Colonoscopy showed: there were polyploidy mucous prominences at hepatic flexure of transverse colon. She did not show any improvement after "hepatic flexure transverse colon polyp resection". The last two months, abdominal pain and other symptoms became further worse, combined with dysuria, urinary pain, and urinary endless. She usually felt a bowel movement coming on, while hard to excrete as dry stool. She started to worry about these symptoms all day long and harder to fall asleep. Laboratory examination: Liver and renal functions, routine blood tests, stool routine test, tumor marker test, abdominal ultrasound were normal. PTC (8-10) 663.6 nmol/L. Examination results of abdominal CT showed that left ureter was mildly dilated, the left renal pelvis had slightly high density, urine salt crystals? Please combine clinical; lymph nodes around the abdominal aorta were slightly increased.The assessment results of WCPA Somatic Symptom Classification Scale for the first time were 0.71 for inhibitory somatic symptoms factor, 2 for irritable somatic symptoms factor, 0 for biological somatic symptoms factor, 2.2 for imaginative somatic symptoms factor, 0.71 for cognitive somatic symptoms factor, the total score 66. He was treated with cymbalta 60mg bid, clonazepam 1mg tid, mosapride 5mg tid, combined with suggestive therapy. 4 week later, the patient reported bloating, bellyache, constipine, dysuria were improved significantly. Second assessment results of WCPA Somatic Symptom Classification Scale were 0.29 for inhibitory somatic symptoms factor, 1 for irritable somatic symptoms factor, 0 for biological somatic symptoms factor, 1.4 for imaginative somatic symptoms factor, 0.43 for cognitive somatic symptoms factor, the total score 36.

Experience: the patient main complaint of bellyache, somatic symptoms scale assessment results show that the imaginative body symptom scores the highest, and imaginative somatic symptoms of pathological psychological foundation is suggested, suggest that closely linked with cognitive function, moreover the second-highest scoring for irritable body symptoms of patients. As mentioned in the first chapter and the second section of this chapter, the imaginary body symptom treatment than other types of physical symptom more individualized and diversified, and the patient's body symptom score higher scores for irritability symptoms, so on the basis of comprehensive treatment, the treatment goals focused on anti-anxiety and symptomatic treatment success.That should be paid attention to by the treatment of the case also is to the body symptoms scale assessment results should be comprehensive analysis, rather than simply only the highest score.

Case 10: on the pathological psychological basis of alexithymia irritable somatic symptoms

Patient zeng , a female , 15 year old, student , with complaint of "vomiting repeatedly for 7 years, recurrence two days ago" . According to the patient's describe , she began to vomit with no obvious inducement 7 years ago , vomiting is a small quantity of stomach contents with no acidity, seizure before the onset of upper abdominal pain with light nausea , without fever , headache and dizziness. Feeling tired and fidget after seizure, eating would exacerbating vomiting. She vomited several times a day, mainly seizure in the daytime, at the beginning, the vomit was small quantity of stomach contents, and then vomited material like water or retching. So she came to digestive system department of local hospital to receive hospitalization, the patient couldn't eat by herself at all during hospital stay, vomited immediately after eating, just kept up primary nutrition by transfusion, with sleep not so deep and easy to weak up, by given general support therapy, symptomatic relieved after a week. After

5months the patient appeared afore-mentioned symptoms again with no obvious inducement, then she received hospitalization at West China Second University Hospital, with nothing wrong with CT, MRI, gastroscope, barium meal, routine examination and so on, the symptoms alleviated by themselves after 7 days. Five months ago, epilepsy after menstruation for two years, three Years ago ictal vomiting appeared again, seizure once every 1-5 months. "Vegetative nerve functional disturbance stomachache" was been diagnosed by other hospital many times, hospitalized and general infusion symptomatic treatment, symptoms will alleviate by themselves in one week, seizure became frequently, the patient's academic record always at the mid but begin to retrogression. She felt anxiety because of this. 2 days ago the patient appear afore-mentioned symptoms again, and come to our hospital.

We diagnosis this patient with anxiety, WCPA Somatic Symptoms Classification Scale were 0.33 for irritable somatic symptoms factor, 0.93 for inhibitory somatic symptoms factor, 0 for biological somatic symptoms factor, 0.7 for imaginative somatic symptoms factor, 0.36 for cognitive somatic symptoms factor. We used Escitalopram 10-20mg/d, olanzapine 2.5mg qn, depakine 500mg qd, clonazepam 1mg bid 2mg qn. After one week's treatment, the patient said that vomiting were gone, anxiety and sleep disorder were obviously improved.and the symptom has not happened again after 1 month, we evaluated again and found that WCPA Somatic Symptoms Classification Scale were 0.08 for irritable somatic symptoms factor, 0.21 for inhibitory somatic symptoms factor, 0 for biological somatic symptoms factor, 0.3 for imaginative somatic symptoms factor, 0 for cognitive somatic symptoms factor. Laboratory examination results: first time the results showed: TSH 1.930mU/L, FT_3 3.60pmol/L, FT_4 20.20pml/L, T_3 0.99nmol/L, T_4 99.47nmol/L, ACTH 76.14ng/L, PTC 397.60nmol/L. After 3 months: TSH 1.930mU/L, FT_3

3.60pmol/L, FT$_4$ 20.20pmol/L, T$_3$ 1.4nmol/L, T$_4$ 99.47nmol/L, ACTH 76.14ng/L, PTC 397.60nmol/L.

Experience: the anxiety of this patient comprehends three aspect, soma aspect — symptoms of organ dysfunction: stomachache, vomit, feeling aspect — agitated, symptoms of sympathetic nervous excitement: palpitation, flustered, cognition aspect — stubborn and inflexible way to think and live, unwilling to change: anxiety.

WCPA Somatic Symptoms Classification Scale show this patient's symptoms as inhibitory somatic symptoms, we used anti-anxiety treatment according to the suggestion of the consensus, and added depakine combined with the biological rhythmic disorders in mood, behavior, sleep and internal secretion.

In the psychological aspect, we can see following ingredients: ①alexithymia: the lost of recognization and expression of emotion cause that she can only express her emotion by soma symptoms. ②obtain benefit: primary obtain benefit can be seen that the patient can escape the hard study, and her mother would not expect too much after she was sick. ③generalized sexual repression: this patient got a standard education since childhood, had a kind of inflexible thinking set and behavior, from this aspect we can understand vomiting as a kind of generalized sexual repression.

(Jing Guo; Zongbin Liao; Jiajia Chen; Cancan Liu; Ting Geng; Ruhan A; Yaling Zhou; Fanmin Zeng; Xueli Sun)

Chapter 5　Conclusion: the consensus

For the above ideas and a series of test and research, the work carried out by the team includes:

a. For the first time, we put forward 4 kinds of classification of somatic symptoms from a comprehensive perspective of psychosomatic medicine; through the development of somatic symptoms classification tools, support more powerful evidence for classification theory hypothesis.

b. Through the empirical study, it is found in the research of direct, psychosomatic medicine, based on the theoretical framework developed by the "WCPA" somatic symptom classification scale of reliability and validity test, the results showed that the self classification tool has good criterion validity, which can be applied to the actual clinical work.

c. Under the theoretical framework of psychosomatic medicine R & D "WCPA Somatic Symptom Classification Scale(R-1) " was a multi-center study, the curative effect of treatment on different somatic symptoms were once again proved that the construction of the theory of this study is scientific and reasonable, the field measurement data are consistent with that of internal structure models. The results of clinical had proved this hypothesis the somatic symptom classification hypothesis reasonable, therefore which can be used in identification of somatic symptoms in clinical practice.

d. The multi-center study proved all the recommended treatment effective on all types of somatic symptoms, it can be used as an important reference in medical practice.

e. Based on the interpretation of the clinical symptom of psychosomatic medicine, in the treatment of chronic non-infectious diseases including at least three dimensions: the first is the etiological treatment, the second is the pathophysiological and pathopsychological dimension, and the third is symptomatic treatment. It shall be noticing that somatic symptoms need more attention.

f. Because of the clinical follow-up time for multi center study is only 3 months. But the 3 months follow-up proved that the treatment effect is market, providing the basis for the theoretical hypothesis for. We will continue to follow up and report on the follow-up results to further verify the hypothesis. In addition, in the questionnaire, the number of subjects is relatively not large enough, mostly from the same working unit. So there may be a selection bias. We will also continue to correct and calibrate the scale to reduce the interference on the results of selective bias.

g. This is the result and summary of research and practice of 2014-2016, the development of formation and the concept is a process of dynamic and continuous falsification, in the process, we will continue to seek the different opinions and expand the scope of practice, and continuously improve the "consensus" which will come in future years.

In a word, the independent treatment of somatic symptoms should be given more attention. Psychosomatic unity and clinical thinking mode of diversification is important to understand somatic symptoms and treatment of somatic symptoms.

(Xueli Sun; Fanmin Zeng)

参考文献/Reference

陈向一，杨德森. 1992. 心身疾病与心身医学. 实用内科学杂志. 1(6)：284-285.

戴晓阳，曹亦薇. 2009. 心理评定量表的编制和修订中存在的一些问题. 中国临床心理学杂志，17(5)：562-565.

范方，耿富磊，张岚，等. 2011. 负性生活事件、社会支持和创伤后应激障碍症状：对汶川地震后青少年的追踪研究. 心理学报，43(12)：1398-1407.

侯永梅. 2004. 心理社会因素对心身疾病的影响. 中国临床康复，8(12)：2358-2359.

孔伶俐，于慧，崔维珍，等. 2014. 躯体形式障碍患者的生活事件和防御方式. 中国健康心理学杂志，22(4)：514-516.

李灿，辛玲. 2008. 调查问卷的信度与效度的评价方法研究. 中国卫生统计，25(5)：541-544.

孙晓娜，李巧莲，陈玉龙. 2003. 生活事件、应付方式和社会支持与胃癌发病的关系. 中国临床康复，7(21)：2954-2955.

孙学礼，曾凡敏. 2015. 临床躯体症状的心身医学分类及诊疗共识，北京：科学出版社.

汪向东，王希林，马弘. 1999. 心理卫生评定量表手册(增订版). 中国心理卫生杂志社. 23-32.

杨放如. 2005. 心身疾病的病因、分类、诊断及其综合防治. 中国医刊，40(7)：57-59.

张向荣，彭昌荣，黄勇孝，等. 2001. 心身疾病患者负性情绪与心理防御机制研究. 健康心理学杂志，9(5)：244.

郑延平，杨德森. 1990. 中国生活事件调查. 中国心理杂志，4(6)：262.

周晓琴，李晓驷，全艳玲，等. 2010. 躯体形式障碍患者的生活事件和应付方式的研究. 精神医学杂志，23(6)：427-428.

Alan R, Laura DK. 2005. Psychologica functioning and physical healh: a paradigm of flexibility. Psychosomatic Medicine. 67, Supplement1: 47-53.

Anderson JC, Gerbin DW. 1988. Structural equation modeling in practice: A review and recommended two step approach. Psychol Bull, 103(3): 411-423.

Arborelius L, Owens MJ, Plotsky PM, et al. 1999. The role of corticotrophin releasing factor in depression and anxiety disorders. J Endocrinol, 160(1): 1-12.

Bagby RM, Parker JDA, Taylor GJ. 1994. The Twenty-Item Toronto Alexithymia Scale: I. Item selection and cross-validation of the factor structure. J Psychosom Res, 38: 23-32.

Bagby RM, Taylor GJ, Parker JDA. 1994. The Twenty-Item Toronto Alexithymia Scale: II. Convergent, discriminant, and concurrent validity. J Psychosom Res, 38: 33-40.

Barsky AJ, Borus JF. 1999. Functional somatic syndromes. Annals of internal medicine, 130(11): 910-921.

Barsky AJ, Peekna HM, Borus JF. 2001. Somatic symptom reporting in women and men. Journal of General Internal Medicine, 16(4): 266-275.

Brenna NR, Leilani F, Daniel LS. 2011. The bidirectional relationship of depression and diabetes: a systematic review. Clinical Psychology Revies, 31: 1239-1246.

Brinholi FF, de Farias CC, Bonifacio KL. 2016. Clozapine and olanzapine are better antioxidants than haloperidol, quetiqpine, risperidone and ziprasidone in in vitro models. Biomedicine & Pharmacotherapy, 81: 411-415.

Brown RJ. 2004. Psychological Mechanisms of medically unexplained symptoms: An Integrative Conceptual Model. Psychological Bulletin, 130(5): 793-812.

Cohen S. 2004. Social relationships and health. Am Psychol, 59(8): 676-684.

Connelly M, Denney DR, 2007. Regulation of emotions during experimental stress in alexithymia. J Psychosom Res, 62: 649-6561.

Costa PT, Jr, McCrae RR. 1992. Revised NEO Personality Inventory (NEO PI-R) and NEO Five-Factor Inventory (NEO-FFI): professional manual. Odessa, FL: Psychological Assessment Resources.

Costa PT, McCrae RR. 1987. Neruoticism, somatic complaints, and disease: is the bark worse than the bite? J Pers, 55: 299-316.

Derbyshire SEG. 1997. Sources of variation in assessing male and female responses to pain. New Ideas Psychol, 15: 83-95.

Derogatis LR, Cleary PA. 1997. Confirmation of the dimensional structure of the SCL-90: A study in construct validation. J Clin Psychol, 33: 981-989.

DeShong HL, Tucker RP, O'Keefe VM, et al. 2015. Five factor model traits as a predictor of suicide ideation and interpersonal suicide risk in a college sampe. Psychiatry Res, 13: S0165-1781.

Eizaguirre AE, Cabezon AOS, Alda IO, et al. 2004. Alexithymia and its relationships with anxiety and depression in eating disorder. Journal of Personality Assessment. 36: 321-331.

Eysenck HJ. 1967. The biological basis of personality. Springfield, IL: Charles C Thomas.

Fabrigar LR, Wegener DT, MacCallum RC, et al. 1999. Evaluating the use of exploratory factor analysis in psychological research. Psychol Methods, 4(3): 272-299.

Fanmin Zeng, Xueli Sun, Bangxiang Yang. 2016. The theoretical construction of a classification of a classification of clinical somatic symptoms in psychosomatic medicine theory. PLOS ONE, 2016. http: // dx. Doi. Org/ 10. 1371/ journal. Pone. 0161222.

Farbod F, Farzaneh N, Bijan MD, et al. 2015. psychological features in patients with and without irritable bowel syndrome: A case-control study using Symptom Checklist-90-REVISED. Indian J Psychiatry. 57(1): 68-72.

Fink P. 1996. Somatization - beyond symptom count. J Psychosom Res, 40 (1) : 7-10.

Fish S. 1967. Organ awareness and organ activation. Psychosom Med. 29: 643-647.

Fred F, Joyce Q. 2007. Alexithymia in Chronic Fatigue Syndrome: Associations With Monentary, Recall, and Retrospective Measures of Somatic Complaints and Emotions.Psychosomatic Medicine. 69: 54-60.

Fukudas Kuratsune H, Tajima S, et al. 2010. Prenorbid personality in chronic fatigue syndrome as determined by the Temperament and Character Inventory. Comprpsychiatry, 51(1): 78-85.

Geisser ME, Roth RS, Theisen ME, et al. 2000. Negative affect, self-report of depression symptoms, and clinical depression: relation to the experience of chronic pain. Clin J Pain, 16: 110-120.

Giovanni AF, Nicoletta S. 2000. Psychosomatic Medicine: Emerging Trends and Perspectives.Psychotherapy and Psychosomatics, 69(4): 184-197.

Hankin BL, Abela, JRZ. 2005. Depression of from childhooh through adolescence and adulthood //Hankin B L, Abela J R Z (Eds.). Development of psychopathology A vulnerability stress perspective. 245-280. New York: SAGE publications. Inc.

Haynes SN, Richard DCS, Kubany ES. 1995. Content validity in psychological assessment: A functional approach to concepts and methods. Psychol Assess, 7(3): 238-247.

Heim C, Ehlert U, Hellhammer DH. 2000. The potential role of hyppcortisolism in the pathophysiology of stress-related bodily disorders. Psychoneuroendocrinology. 25(1): 1-35.

Hong J, Novick D, Montgomery W. Real-world outcomes in patients with depression treated with duloxetine or a selective serotonin reuptake inhibitor in East Asia. Asia-Pacific psychiatry, 2016, 8(1): 51-59.

Hotop FM. 2004. Preventing somatization. Psychol Med, 34: 195-198.

James F. Reed III. 2000. Homogeneity of kappa statistics in multiple samples. Computer Methods and Programs in Biomedicine, 63: 43-46.

Strain JJ. 1979. The relationship between psychoanalysis and psychosomatic medicine. Psyccritiques . 24, 11.

Jiri H, Erik H, Iveta N. 2000. Treatment of Interictal Depression with Citalopram in Patients with Epilepsy. Epilepsy & Behavior: 444-447.

Johnson-Kozlow MF, Sallis JF, Calfas KJ. 2004. Does life stress moderate the effects of a physical activity intervention? Psychol Health, 19(4): 479-489.

Katon W, Kleinman A, Rosen G. 1982. Depression and somatization: A review: Part

I. Am J Med, 72: 127-135.

Katon W, Kleinman A, Rosen G. 1982. Depression and somatization: A review: Part II. Am J Med, 72: 241-247.

Kirmayer LJ, Robbins JM, Dworkind M, et al. 1993. Somatization and the recognition of depression and anxiety in primary care. Am J Psychiatry, 150: 734-741.

Kolk AM, Gijsbers CM, Van Vliet KP, et al. 1991. Symptom sensitivity and sex differences in physical morbidity: a review of health surveys in the United States and the Netherlands. Women Health, 17: 91-124.

Kroenke K, Spitzer R, Williams JBW. 2002. The PHQ-15: Validity of a new measure for evaluating the severity of somatic symptoms. Psychosom Med, 64(2): 258-266.

Lakshmi NY. 2011. A clinical review of aripiprazole in bipolar depression and maintance therapy of bipolar disorder. Journal of Affective Disorders, 128SI: S21-S28.

Lawton MP. 1959. The screening value of the Cornell Medical Index. J Consult Psychol, 23(4): 352-356.

Leserman J, Drossman DA. 1995. Sexual and physical abuse history and medical practice. Gen Hosp Psychiatry, 17: 71-74.

Li Dm, Zheng J, Wang My. 2016. Wuling powder prevents the depression-like behavior in learned helplessness mice model through improving the TSPO mediated-mitophagy. Journal of Ethnopharmacology, 186, 181-188.

Linzer M, Spitzer R, Kroenke K, et al. 1996. Gender, quality of life, and mental disorders in primary care: results from the PRIME-MD 1000 study. AM J Med, 101: 526-533.

Lipowsk ZJ. Wha Does the Word "Psychosomatic" Really Mean? A Historical and Semantic Inquiry. Psychosomatic Medicine. 1984, 46(2): 153-171.

Lipsitt DR. 1982. The painful woman: complaints, symptoms, and illness. In: Notman MT, Nadelson CC, eds. Women in Context: The Women Patient. New York: Plenum, 147-152.

Liu XC, Dai ZS, Tang MQ, et al. 1994. Factor analysis of Self-Rating Depression

Scale (SDS). Chin J Clin Psychol, 3: 151-154.

Liu XH, Li T. 2010. Oxford textbook of psychiatry. 5th ed. Chengdu: Sichuan University Press.

MacCallum RC, Austin JT. 2000. Applications of structural equation modeling in psychological research. Ann Rev Psychol, 51: 201-226.

Mechanic D. 1972. Social psychologic factors affecting the presentation of bodily complaints. New Engl J Med, 285: 1132-1139.

Merskey H, DM. 1997. Response to Editorial: New perspectives on the Definition of Pain. Pain, 67(1): 209.

Miller GE, Chen E, Zhou ES. 2007. If it goes up, must it come down? Chronic stress and the hypothalamic-pituitary-adrenocortical axis in humans. Psychol Bull, 133: 25-45.

Oddone CG, Hybels CF, McQuoid D, et al. 2011. Social support modifies the relationship between personality and depressive symptoms in older adults. The Americal Journal of Geriatric Psychiatry, 19(2): 123-131.

Ouyang QIN., Wu H, Liu C. 2010. Clinical diagnostics. 2nd ed . (7-11): Beijing: People's Medical Publishing House Press.

Pannell J. 2009. Suggestive interventions in psychoanalysis. Am J Psychoanal. 69(3): 263-5.

Pariante CM, Miller AH. 2001. Glucocortcoid receptors in major depression: relevance to pathophysiology and treatment. Biol Psychiatry, 49(5): 391-404.

Parker JDA, Taylor GJ, Bagby RM. 2003. The 20-Item Toronto Alexithymia Scale: III. Reliability and factorial validity in a community population. J Psychosom Res, 55: 269-275.

Patel V, Kirkwood BR, Weiss H, 2005. Chronic fatigue in developing countries: population based survey of women in India. BMJ, 330(7501): 1190.

Ray C, Lindop J. 1982. The Concept of Coping. Psychological Medicine, 1: 385-395.

Richard DL. 2008. Neural Substrates of Implicit and Explicit Emotional Processes: A Unifying Framework for Psychosomatic Medicine. Psychosomatic Medicine. 70:

214-231.

Rief W, Mewes R, Martin A, et al. 2010. Are psychological features useful in classifying patients with somatic symptoms? Psychosom Med, 72: 648-655.

Saariaho AS, Sarriaho TH, Mattila AK, et al. 2013. Alexithymia and depression in a chronic pain patient sample. Gen Hosp Psychiatry, 35: 239-245.

Sarason JG. 1978. Assessing the impact of Life change: development of life experiences survey J of consulting and clinical Psychology, 46: 932.

Silverstein B, Blumenthal E. 1997. Depression mixed with anxiety, somatization and disordered eating: relationships with gender role- related limitations experienced by females. Sex Roles. 36: 709-724.

Streiner DL. 1994. Figuring out factors: The use and misuse of factor analysis. Canadian Journal of Psychiatr, 39: 135-140.

Stuart AM, David S B, Pierre B. 2007. Which antidepressants have demonstrated superior efficacy? A review of the evidence. International Clinical Psychopharmacology, 22(6): 323-329.

Sumiyoshi T, Matsui, M, Yamashita I. 2000. Effect of Adjunctive Treatment With Serotonin-1A Aonist Tandospirone on Memory Functions in Schizophrenia. Journal of Clinical Psychopharmacology, 20(3): 386-388.

Sun X. 2013. Enlightenment from common somatic symptoms of clinical depression. Chin J Psychiatry, 46: 371-372.

Taylor G. 2000. Recent developments in alexithymia theory and research. Can J Psychiatry. 45: 134-142.

Taylor GJ, Bagby RM, Parker JDA. 2003. The Twenty-Item Toronto Alexithymia Scale: IV. Reliability and factorial validity in different languages and cultures. J Psychosom Res, 55: 277-283.

Uchino BN. 2006. Social support and health: a review of physiological processes potentially underlying links to disease outcomes. J Behav Med, 29(4): 377-387.

VanderWeide LA, Smith SM, Trinkley KE. 2015. Asystematic review of the efficacy of venlafaxine for the treatment of fibromyalgia. Journal of Clinical Pharmacy and

Therapeutics, 40: 1-6.

Verbrugge LM. 1980. Sex differences in complaints and diagnoses. Behav Med, 3: 327-355.

Vignola RC, Tucci AM. 2014. Adaptation and validation of the depression, anxiety and stress scale (DASS) to Brazilian Portuguese. J Affect Disord, 155: 104-109.

Waller E. 2004. Somatoform disorders as disorders of affect regulation A study comparing the TAS-20 with monself report measures of alexithymia. J Psychosom Res, 57(3): 239-247.

Wang X, Wang X, Ma H. 1999. Rating scales for mental health. Rev ed, Beijing: Xinhua Publishing House. 23-32.

Wang ZY. 1984. Chinese version of Zung's self-rating anxiety scale. Shanghai Arch Psychiatry, 2: 73-74.

Warner CD. 1995. Somatic awareness and coronary artery disease in women with chest pain. Heart Lung, 24: 436-443.

Waston D, Pennebaker JW. 1989. Health complaint stress and distress Exploring the central role of negative affectivity. Psychol Rey, 96(2): 234-254.

Williams, PG, O'Brien, CD, Colder, CR. 2004. The effects of neuroticism and extraversion on self-assessed health and health-relevant cognition. Personality Individual Difference, 37: 83-94.

Willian JG, David TG. 1952. Relationship of Specific Attitudes and Emotions to Certain Bodily Diseases. Psychosomatic Medicine. 4: 243-251.

Yan XJ, Li WT, Wang EM. 2015. Effect of Clinician-patient communication on compliance with flupentixol-melitracen in functional dyspepsia patients. World J Gastroenterol 21(15): 4652-4659.

Zhang X, Kang D, Zhang L. 2014. Shuganjieyu capsule for major depressive disorder(MDD) in adults: a systematic review. Aging & Mental Health, 18(8): 941-953.